RX FOR HOPE

RX FOR HOPE

An Integrative Approach to Cancer Care

Nick Chen, MD
and
David Tabatsky

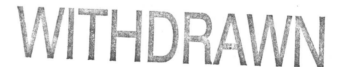

ROWMAN & LITTLEFIELD
Lanham • Boulder • New York • London

Published by Rowman & Littlefield
An imprint of The Rowman & Littlefield Publishing Group, Inc.
4501 Forbes Boulevard, Suite 200, Lanham, Maryland 20706
www.rowman.com

Unit A, Whitacre Mews, 26-34 Stannary Street, London SE11 4AB

British Library Cataloguing in Publication Information Available

Library of Congress Cataloging-in-Publication Data Available

ISBN: 978-1-5381-0160-5 (cloth : alk. paper)
ISBN: 978-1-5381-0161-2 (electronic)

Printed in the United States of America

CONTENTS

ACKNOWLEDGMENTS

I want to acknowledge all my patients whose courage and intuition about life were the inspiration of my work in the first place. I want to thank all the staff at Seattle Integrative Cancer Center who create a warm, supportive environment for our patients and enable my work to be as smooth as possible.

I also want to thank my coauthor, David Tabatsky, and my agent, Nancy Rosenfeld—without their perseverance and encouragement this book would not be possible. Thanks to Suzanne Staszak-Silva and staff at Rowman & Littlefield for editorial support. I want to give special thanks to Mr. Bruce Watson, a seven-year survivor of advanced pancreatic cancer whose story is in this book, and who also provided additional editorial work for this book while on chemotherapy.

I want to dedicate this book to my father, who passed away two and a half years ago. His deep knowledge of human immunology and his unfailing spirit of scientific inquisition still influence me today.

Finally, thanks to my wife, Lucia, and children, Emily and Kenny, who make my life complete.

—Nick Chen, MD, PhD
Seattle, WA

My thanks to Nick Chen, his staff, and the many wonderful patients he serves so beautifully who I have been fortunate to meet in Seattle. Thanks to our agent, Nancy Rosenfeld (and to the memory of her dear friend,

Jean-Yves Pavée). Thanks to Suzanne Staszak-Silva and her colleagues at Rowman & Littlefield.

I wish this book had been around to help my father, and so many others I miss. Jan, Jeff, Nils, Bob, Dani, Linn, Claudia, Samuel, Jamie, and Rick—this is for you.

—David Tabatsky
New York City

INTRODUCTION

Redefining Hope with a Commonsense, Integrative Approach to Cancer Care

After receiving a terminal diagnosis of colon cancer in 2005, Richard underwent multiple rounds of conventional radiation and chemotherapy treatments at a series of large cancer centers, but his tumors did not respond and metastasized. Richard became a "cancer refugee," searching the Pacific Northwest for options. Eventually he found us. My team and I were able to change what was once a death sentence into an ongoing journey of life sustaining treatments.

Ellen was diagnosed in 2002 with stage 4 lung cancer. She was told she had barely nine months to live and that her only hope was high-dose chemotherapy. Like Richard, she could not accept such a dismal prognosis and began a search for a more hopeful approach. When she eventually found us, she opted to follow my protocol of metronomic low-dose chemotherapy, along with the rebuilding of her immune system with diet, nutrition, and supplements. By the end of 2003, her tumor had shrunk into complete remission. She has maintained her health by following our integrative approach over the past fifteen years, and recently celebrated her eighty-ninth birthday with her family.

After surgery for prostate cancer in 2010, Robert was diagnosed a year later with aggressive stage 4 mantle cell lymphoma. Three different doctors agreed that the only option for Robert was a stem cell transplant, which *might* give him an additional five years, with likely relapses. They added that he probably would live for a year at most if he did not undergo the transplantation procedure. After meeting with us through a referral, Robert chose to follow our recommendation of receiving weekly low doses of chemotherapy, along with high-dose intravenous vitamin C and other dietary changes and supplements, for twenty-four weeks. This treatment resulted in complete remission that has now lasted over seven years. In response to these developments, Robert said, "This was the first time I had any hope after being treated in multiple institutions like a number."

By conventional medical standards, there is no reason Richard, Ellen, or Robert should still be with us. They are thus living proof of the efficacy of the integrative approach to cancer care that our care team and I provide at the Seattle Integrative Cancer Center. They exemplify how low-dose metronomic chemotherapy and immunotherapy can boost the immune system and control cancer, effectively turning it into a manageable, long-term chronic illness.

These three patients, like hundreds of others we have treated, are the rule, not the exception. They demonstrate how a gentle and commonsense approach to cancer treatment—both short- and long-term—can produce consistent results that conventional treatments often cannot. It's about hope and using the best of what science has to offer to harness the power of the immune system for cancer control.

Our integrative approach is qualitatively different from the way cancer has traditionally been treated. From my experience over the last fifteen plus years as an oncologist with a PhD in immunology, I have become convinced that the welfare of the immune system holds the key for success in all cancer treatments.

Considering the current state of medicine and the challenges of treating cancer, we are doing our patients a grave disservice by maintaining the status quo of conventional treatments. Despite the progress being made in research laboratories, conventional wisdom—especially when it comes to the model of maximally tolerated dose chemotherapy with disregard of patients' general wellness—must be challenged if we are ever going to improve the status of cancer care in this country from the perspective of patients.

America's fascination with drugs never gets old. From aspirin for a simple headache to medicines for a depressed mood, we look to pills and shots to fix our bodies, no matter what the root cause may be.

Unfortunately, this approach also applies to the world of cancer, where most well-meaning oncologists inevitably prescribe chemotherapy—and lots of it—even though cancer is a complicated disease requiring a multifaceted approach. It is now clear that cancer is affected by such factors as the interaction of mind and body, interaction between a tumor and its biological microenvironment, diet, nutrition, emotional well-being, and exercise. All of these factors influence the biology of cancer and the ability of the immune system to fight it.

As a long-standing member of the American Medical Association, the American Board of Internal Medicine and Medical Oncology, and the American Society of Clinical Oncology, I am quite familiar with today's status quo in treating cancer. As a participating member of the Society for Integrative Oncology and the Oncology Association of Naturopathic Physicians, I am also an active participant in the ongoing discussion about complementary and alternative cancer treatments.

Over the last fifteen years, my colleagues and I have developed a gentler but more consistent form of chemotherapy called metronomic low-dose chemotherapy (MLDC) for most types of cancer we treat in our practice. This methodology is both significantly more effective and better tolerated. We combine this with a nourishing array of integrative medicine that further reduces patients' treatment side effects, boosts their immune systems, and improves their quality of life. In the end, we have created a model of cancer care that has produced treatment outcomes unmatchable by the current conventional cancer care standard and its statistics.

At the Seattle Integrative Cancer Center, we strive to keep our patients and their inner healing power at the center of our care. We enlist patients as our partners in building up an alliance of science, medicine, nature's healing power, and common sense to overcome cancer and restore life's balance. We educate our patients about their cancer and rational ways to treat them. We emphasize the immune system as the most important player in achieving the long-term control of cancer. We teach our patients how to maintain and enhance their immune system while promoting a genuinely hopeful and holistic atmosphere of healing. This emphasis on guiding our patients toward an integrative cancer treatment that encompasses every aspect of the healing process is one of the major factors that set us apart. The feedback from our patients, expressing high satisfaction with the care they receive and the excitement of achieving great treatment results, has been a steady reinforcement for our belief in the superiority of this care model. It is also our motivation for writing this book—to share this knowledge with more patients who need it for their life.

This is the essence of *Rx for Hope*.

This "common sense" approach, focusing on the evident role of the immune system in cancer control, is the foundation of our integrative model. Its position is grounded between holistic and precision medicine. By contrast, traditional cancer care still defers to obsolete "carpet bombing" methods when it comes to prescribing maximally tolerated doses of chemotherapy or with "targeted therapy" that is so restricted in efficacy scope that it is akin to the adage of "see the tree but miss the forest." Those of us who take a more open-minded approach face skepticism and even ridicule when we stress the importance of our inner healing power in cancer control and the benefits of supporting it through commonsense lifestyle changes and science-backed complementary medicine during cancer treatment. But time may have proven us right, as more and more medicine aimed at boosting immune response to cancer have raced into markets. Although these developments are a proof of principle, our emphasis on the day-to-day integrative medicine action that conditions our bodies and strengthens our immune systems is irreplaceable with any man-made drugs. Additionally, these immunotherapy agents are not going to work well with the conventional immunosuppressive high-dose chemotherapy and, unless the latter is changed, the cancer treatment outcome will remain disappointing for the majority of patients.

Rx for Hope presents convincing scientific evidence and extensive clinical experience that supports a way to administer chemotherapy that is both safer and more effective than the standard method. This book explores the scientific origin of low-dose chemotherapy—also known as metronomic chemotherapy—and discusses the mechanisms that can be further enhanced by a menu of complementary integrative medicine. It compares low-dose to high-dose chemotherapy, particularly in relation to their difference in influencing the anticancer immune response and cancer's microenvironment. It lays out a logical, detailed, and easy-to-read argument for the benefits of a more holistic, integrative approach to the way we heal people with cancer and set them on a path of better health.

The validity of this approach is also backed up by over fifteen years of clinical experience and research, as well as by many patient profiles from the Seattle Integrative Cancer Center that are described throughout the book.

The current cancer treatment system, while improving patients' survival sometimes, almost invariably decreases patients' quality of life; this clearly indicates that a different and more comprehensive approach is needed. *Rx for Hope* also discusses the abundant evidence that our psychological function, physical activity, and the food we eat can affect us at detailed biological levels, all the way to our DNA, where they can alter gene expression and change how our body reacts to the presence of cancer. Therefore, cancer treatment benefits from options beyond the use of conventional drugs. It presents a treatment-supporting integrative approach based on scientific evidence and discusses how they can complement our core treatment methods.

Recent years have witnessed the exciting development of a new modality of cancer treatment—immunotherapy. Not only is it a proof of principle to what we believe, it provides our patients with alternative treatments that we didn't have before. *Rx for Hope* discusses many ways our integrative model of care provides the perfect foundation to integrate these new treatment methods. By reviewing the benefits and limitations of these treatments, we explore how we can overcome their deficiency and enhance their efficacy by combining them with our integrative therapies. How these interventions converge—inducing a powerful antitumor immune response—is the key to lasting cancer control.

It is bitterly ironic that, even in this era in which new cancer drugs and therapies emerge virtually every month, we also see a stagnation of outcomes in terms of survival and quality of life. This stagnation is due to the fact new therapies are only benefiting a minority of lucky patients and that most cancer patients are still dependent on old fundamentally defective chemotherapy methods that are both toxic and ineffective.

This reality is likely to last a long time if no changes are made in the treatment paradigm. And while new cancer drugs are becoming more precise or targeted, less attention is being paid to the overall health and well-being of the patient. Ignoring this is profoundly wrongheaded if the goal is long-term cancer control and improving a patient's quality of life.

Recent scientific findings and the successful experiences that we see at our clinic demonstrate an urgent need to reevaluate the current conventional approach to cancer treatment. We strongly endorse a progressive treatment model, combining metronomic low-dose chemotherapy with complementary integrative medicine. Combined with new, breakthrough immunotherapy drugs, these treatments have the potential to create a response powerful enough to eradicate detectable cancer as well as prevent its recurrence.

Every twenty-three seconds someone in America is diagnosed with cancer, and the number of people affected is growing rapidly. The American Cancer Society estimates that nearly 2 million *new* patients will need treatment in the coming year. On the basis of current trends and methods of treatment, far too many of these people will be treated *without* the benefits of metronomic low-dose chemotherapy, and even less will enjoy the positive impact of immune-supportive, complementary integrative medicine. Most of these patients would experience better outcomes if we expanded the toolbox of medical professionals and provided an educational blueprint for patients.

The medical revolution we advocate begins with a pragmatic approach and the emotional and spiritual energy of hope. This speaks directly to the main purpose of this book, which is to let patients know about treatment options that they can explore. This applies to newly diagnosed patients as well as to those whose current treatment is not yielding satisfying results, especially patients for whom conventional treatments have failed but who are not yet ready to give up.

Another reason for this book is to open a discussion with oncologists and others within the cancer community about the success of a treatment model combining low-dose, metronomic chemotherapy with integrative medicine. Admittedly, this is not something that can be easily tested by a randomized placebo-controlled double-blind study. However, if the model is studied as a whole and its outcome data collected based on all the integrative care provided, it will easily demonstrate its superiority to conventional care. Anyone who patiently studies this model with an open mind will find it to be a commonsense approach that isn't hard to understand. Our hope is that more and more people will discover the value of this comprehensive approach and begin using it to their comfort level. I am sure that they will soon have a taste of the success that we are experiencing on a daily basis.

Rx for Hope is novel in that it brings together two complementing cancer treatment methods—metronomic low-dose chemotherapy and complementary medicine—and creates a convincing case for an ideal cancer treatment model that is backed by both science and years of real-life experience. While bookstores and websites contain some titles covering either of these topics, none really discusses the combined model or explores the synergy to such a depth. It is particularly suitable for patients with conventionally treatable cases who strongly prefer a gentler, holistic approach. It would be a much better option for them than just completely going "alternative" when traditional treatments have failed. The methods described in this book will provide patients with new hope in a new direction. Indeed, for anyone facing a cancer diagnosis of any kind, the integrative approach will not only be unique; it might well be a lifesaver.

If you are a cancer patient, caregiver, and/or survivor, keep reading. If you are a medical student or oncology professional, you may be looking for new insights to the traditional treatments you have learned, especially those that continue to disappoint because of their lack of enduring success. If any of these descriptions fit your situation, *Rx for Hope* is for you.

I feel fortunate each and every day to be serving Richard, Ellen, Robert, and all of my patients and their families, who continue to see the steady results of combining the best of all sciences to serve them. I hope you will find inspiration, as I have, from these wonderful stories, as well as from an abundance of new information to help you participate in a better system of cancer care.

By educating patients about possibilities and options, as well as opening the minds of conventional oncologists willing to explore new treatment strategies, we are taking bold steps toward improving the life for cancer patients everywhere.

Finally, we may soon be able to declare that cancer has become a chronic disease, like heart disease, diabetes, or even lupus, a disease that our patients can manage and live with successfully. We firmly believe that the methodologies presented in *Rx for Hope* will help us get there faster.

1

FROM MUSTARD GAS TO MODERN MEDICINE

The Origins, Evolution, and Efficacy of Maximum Tolerated Dose (MTD) Chemotherapy

A mysterious cloud of shiny dust hovered over Allied troops fighting in World War I in Belgium during the summer of 1917. Suddenly, soldiers were overcome by a peppery smell and experienced terrible itching and burning on their skin and started to cough uncontrollably. The silvery dust was mustard gas, and it created a level of torture never seen before on any battlefield. The era of chemical warfare had dawned.

Ironically, this poisonous gas later led to the discovery of the first effective cancer-killing drug, nitrogen mustard, and a very different type of war, one fought in a laboratory instead of a battlefield.

THE ORIGINS OF MODERN CHEMOTHERAPY

German scientist and physician Paul Ehrlich (1854–1915) initially coined the term *chemotherapy* in 1909 after he discovered arsphenamine, the first chemical-based drug which, a year later, became the first effective treatment for syphilis.

Ehrlich also helped popularize the idea of a "magic bullet" in treating human diseases, an idea that still influences physicians and scientists treating cancer today. He later became famous as the first person to document the effectiveness of animal models to screen a series of chemicals for their potential activity against diseases.

Ehrlich was also interested in drugs to treat cancer, including aniline dyes, one of the first primitive alkylating agents. Interestingly, he was not so optimistic about the chance of success right from the beginning. In fact, the laboratory where he conducted this work had a sign over the door that read "Give up all hope, oh ye who enter."

Early treatment of cancer was dominated by surgery, which focused primarily on removing tumors, along with any surrounding tissues that may have been affected. This approach reflected the early observation that cancer is an aggressive tissue-invading disease, and that removing *only* the visible tumor would have minimal benefit for the patient. Although doctors treating cancer at this time quickly realized that many resected cancers would return in a location far from the original tumor, they had no means of preventing or treating these recurrences. Moreover, some cancers, such as lymphoma and leukemia, are just not treatable with surgery alone.

EARLY CANCER DRUG DEVELOPMENT

The understanding from Paul Ehrlich's work in the early twentieth century that certain chemicals can kill cancer was followed by more studies on different chemicals that might affect the disease. The discovery of these early chemotherapeutic drugs continued into the 1940s. Most of this work depended on the use of transplantable tumor models in rodents to screen for useful chemicals for human use. George Clowes, of Roswell Park Memorial Institute in Buffalo, New York, developed the first transplantable tumor systems in rodents in 1910. This advance prompted the standardization of model systems and the testing of larger numbers of chemicals. Subsequent work focused on identifying the ideal model system for cancer drug testing, which became a major thrust of research for the next several decades. Murray Shear, who later became known to his colleagues at the National Institutes of Health as "the father of chemotherapy," set up a collaborative program that would become a model for cancer drug screening in 1935. This program was the first to test a broad array of compounds, including natural products. However, no breakthrough in the finding of the first cancer treatment drug occurred until mustard gas emerged again in the midst of World War II.

WORLD WAR II AND THE POSTWAR PERIOD

Although gases were not used on the battlefield in World War II, the observation that soldiers exposed to mustard gas leaked from a bombed ship in Bari Harbor, Italy, had depleted numbers of certain immune cells called lymphocytes led scientists to speculate that mustard gas might help patients with cancer from the lymphoid system.

Scientists Milton Winternitz, Alfred Gilman, and Louis Goodman from Yale University partnered with the U.S. Office of Scientific Research and Development to study the chemistry of mustard compounds to determine if these chemicals might have valuable therapeutic effects in cancer treatment.[1] Winternitz, then the dean of the Yale University Medical School, had studied the use of sulfur mustards during World War I, and Gilman and Goodman were both well-respected pharmacologists. They transplanted lymphoid tumors into mice and then injected them with nitrogen mustard, a stable compound derived from mustard gas. After observing regressions of the tumors in mice, these same scientists, working with Dr. Gustaf Lindskog, a colleague and thoracic surgeon, identified a human patient with advanced lymphoma. This patient—referred to simply as JD—had a large tumor on his jaw and could not swallow or sleep. The lymph nodes under his arms were so inflamed that he could barely fold his arms across his chest. His doctors had tried every treatment they had at their disposal, but nothing had affected the tumor. JD's prognosis was bleak, and since he had nothing to lose, he agreed to try the experimental nitrogen mustard that had caused tumor regression in mice.

One morning in August 1942, JD received an injection of a synthetic lymphocidal chemical, the nitrogen mustard used to make mustard gas. With the war raging and controversy surrounding the use of chemical warfare, JD's case was kept secret. He received several treatments with what was referred to as "substance X." These treatments soon allowed him to sleep, swallow, and eat.

Unfortunately, JD's cancer relapsed and he died six months after receiving the treatment, unaware that his participation in the experiment had ushered in a new era of cancer treatment—the use of chemotherapy.[2]

Across the Atlantic, work done over the following years by a brilliant chemist, Professor Alexander Haddow, led to the landmark *Nature* publication in 1948 that described the chemical structure responsible for the cancer-killing effect of nitrogen mustard, and paved the way for the future development of safer and more effective cancer treatment drugs.

The pharmaceutical industry became involved in another World War II–related program when it undertook a large-scale screening of fermentation products to isolate and produce antibiotics to treat infections. These studies were influenced by the possibility of antitumor effects in certain agents found in penicillin. One such agent, the antibiotic actinomycin D, came out of this program. Actinomycin D was found to have significant antitumor properties and was frequently used to treat pediatric tumors in the 1950s and 1960s. The discovery of this drug sparked the initial interest in searching for more active antitumor antibiotics and led to the discovery of a number of active antitumor antibiotics such as adriamycin, that are still in common use.

In 1955, more than twenty-five years after the completion of four World War II–related science programs, the effects of the drugs that evolved from them triggered the establishment of a national drug development effort known as the Cancer Chemotherapy National Service Center (CCNSC). Today, more than two hundred cancer treatment drugs listed from A to Z on the National Cancer Institute (NCI) website are available for treating a variety of cancers.

THE EVOLUTION OF MODERN CHEMOTHERAPY

As defined by the American Cancer Society (ACS), chemotherapy "usually refers to the use of medicines or drugs to treat cancer," and is used to "keep the cancer from spreading, slow the cancer's growth, kill cancer cells that may have spread to other parts of the body, and to relieve symptoms, such as pain or blockages, caused by cancer."

Doctor Sidney Farber, after whom the Dana-Farber Cancer Institute of Harvard Medical School is named, was the pioneer in using chemotherapy to treat leukemia, a cancer of blood-producing cells. While working as a pathologist at Harvard's Children's Hospital, he led both preclinical and clinical studies of aminopterin, a folate antagonist (a substance that interferes with the action of folic acid or "folate"), in the treatment of acute childhood lymphoblastic leukemia.

While folate is a nutrient that promotes the proliferation of leukemic cells, aminopterin competitively inhibits internal folate synthesis, which leads to the arrest of DNA and RNA synthesis of the leukemic cells. In a publication in the *New England Journal of Medicine* in 1948, Farber showed for the first time that the administration of aminopterin could cause both clinical and hematological remissions, even though the remissions were temporary. Subsequently, researchers developed similar drugs that blocked other cellular functions, and these breakthroughs have gradually expanded the landscape of modern-day chemotherapy. Today, acute lymphoblastic leukemia is one of the most curable human malignancies, with about a 90 percent cure rate ten years after diagnosis.

By 1951, two drugs were in development, 6-thioquanine and 6-mercaptopurine, both of which would eventually play an important role in treating acute leukemia. But it was not until the middle 1950s that drugs were developed targeting nonhematologic cancers (cancers that do not target blood cells).

In 1856, cancer researcher Charles Heidelberger, who studied the DNA/RNA synthesis of tumor cells at the University of Wisconsin, developed the first pyrimidine analogue, named 5-fluorouracil (5-FU), that can competitively inhibit the tumor DNA synthesis by attaching a fluorine atom to the 5-position of the uracil pyrimidine base. This agent demonstrated broad-spectrum activity against a range of solid tumors and remains a cornerstone for treating multiple cancers, including colon, gastric, and breast cancers.[3]

We could say that this represents the first use of what we now call *targeted therapy*, a primary focus in developing today's cancer drugs, even though the original target was a biochemical pathway and not a molecular target. These breakthroughs in developing anticancer drugs spurred interest in chemotherapy. As a result, laboratories sprung up to study more tumors in mice, leading to a series of independent screening programs all over the world.

Postwar science and drug development found many homes in America, but the largest and perhaps the most influential was located in New York City at the Sloan-Kettering Institute (SKI). Under the leadership of

Cornelius "Dusty" Rhoads, most of the personnel from the Chemical Warfare Service, including David Karnofsky, a pioneer in clinical investigation, were brought into the drug development program at SKI.

Dr. Rhoads and his team used the murine (mouse) S180 model as their primary screening tool, while researchers in other hospitals chose other models. Although there were only a handful of facilities devoted to testing clinical drugs for patients at this time, there were a number of locations in which such research flourished. Among these hotbeds of research were the Children's Cancer Research Foundation in Boston, under Sydney Farber; the Southern Research Institute in Birmingham, Alabama, under Howard Skipper; Japan's largest cancer center; and the Chester Beatty Research Institute in London, under the guidance of Alexander Haddow.

In 1954, the Senate Appropriations Committee provided $1 million— a relatively ample sum at the time—for cancer drug development, which unleashed a tribal battle for how those funds would be spent. Congress eventually upped their support, giving the National Cancer Institute (NCI) $5 million and a mandate to establish the Cancer Chemotherapy National Service Center (CCNSC). The establishment of the CCNSC entailed setting up a structure to work discreetly with commercial interests, creating access to clinical testing facilities, making resources available for pharmacology and toxicology testing and drug production, and formulating a system to ensure that drugs met specific criteria at every point in their creation and use. One of the more important activities was the creation of a series of committees that were tasked with the development of hormone therapy, the development of statistical analyses to assess drug efficacy, the development of protocols to administer drugs, and the design and conduct of clinical trials. Many of the procedures developed by these committees in the 1950s are still in use today.

Although it was often criticized, the CCNSC enabled the birth of a multibillion-dollar cancer pharmaceutical industry. It provided a centralized clearinghouse to test, develop, and produce drugs, as well as clinical studies that could not have happened on their own in academic circles or within the pharmaceutical industry.

The first concrete evidence that chemotherapy could effectively treat advanced solid tumors occurred in 1958, when Chinese-American physician and cancer researcher Dr. Min Chiu Li used methotrexate, a drug derived from aminopterin, to eradicate a very rare tumor of the placenta (choriocarcinoma). Li was subsequently credited as the first physician to use chemotherapy to cure metastatic, malignant cancer.

Born in China, Li studied at Mukden Medical College, in present-day Shenyang. He came to the United States in 1947 for medical training at the University of Southern California and, because of the Chinese Revolution, was unable to return to his homeland. After residencies at Chicago's Presbyterian Hospital (now Rush University Medical Center) and Memorial Hospital in New York City (now Memorial Sloan-Kettering Cancer Center), he became obsessed with finding a cure for cancer. This desire was fueled by witnessing patients endure terrible suffering as they died from choriocarcinoma.

Li began treating his choriocarcinoma patients with an antifolate chemotherapy drug called methotrexate. Although he and his colleagues were unable to demonstrate any improvement in patient health, they found that when patients were being treated with methotrexate, urine levels of the hormone human chorionic gonadotropin (hCG) dropped steadily. Li hypothesized that the patients' tumors were secreting hCG. If this were so, the level of hCG in a patient's urine could be used to measure the effectiveness of a particular treatment, the same concept of cancer tumor marker testing nowadays.

In 1955, after moving to the National Cancer Institute, Li tested his hypotheses on a twenty-four-year-old woman who had developed metastatic choriocarcinoma lesions in her lungs. When one of the lesions ruptured, her chest cavity filled with blood and air, leaving her in grave condition. Li administered a single 10 mg dose of methotrexate. Against all odds, she survived through the next day, at which point Li administered a 50 mg dose. Over the next several days, her hCG levels decreased slightly, but soon they became elevated again. Li decided to try four daily doses of 25 mg. The patient improved enough that within three weeks she was able to sit up in a chair. Li repeated the regimen of daily doses and, although she suffered from several complications brought on by the toxicity of the drugs, including low blood cell counts, diarrhea, and stomatitis, the patient continued to improve.

Within four months, Li's patient exhibited no evidence of disease. In continuing his success in using methotrexate to treat patients with choriocarcinoma in the lungs, Dr. Li and his colleagues made two important observations.[4] First, they found that drug-dosing schedules have a strong effect on efficacy. Patients treated with 125 mg of methotrexate daily for four to five days had better outcomes than patients treated with one large dose of methotrexate just once. Second, patients who were treated until the tumor disappeared *and* their urinary hCG levels normalized were cured, whereas those treated only until the tumor disappeared invariably experienced a recurrence.

Ironically, Dr. Li was fired by the NCI for treating choriocarcinoma patients to hCG normalization because he was being perceived as causing unnecessary toxicity to patients by administering unnecessary additional chemotherapy. He was, however, vindicated when later studies proved he was right. Indeed, fellow cancer researcher Emil Freireich considered Li's insight that tumors with chemical markers would recur unless treated until the marker had normalized to be an "extraordinarily important new principle in cancer treatment."[5] Before Li's work, over 90 percent of patients diagnosed with choriocarcinoma died within a year. Now, nearly all patients diagnosed with choriocarcinoma can be cured with chemotherapy alone.

Li went on to develop the first effective combination chemotherapy program for metastatic testicular cancer in 1970. He won the prestigious Lasker-DeBakey Clinical Research Award for his work in 1972.

CHANGING THE PARADIGM OF CARE

The notion of using chemotherapy as an effective treatment for cancer opened many minds throughout the medical world. Because combination chemotherapy cured some types of rarer but advanced cancers, such as choriocarcinoma and testicular cancer, oncologists hoped that the same results could be achieved for the more common, solid tumors in early stage diseases. The adjuvant chemotherapy concept was initially tested in breast and colon cancers.

Breast cancer treatment was dominated in the early days by radical mastectomy, sometimes called the Halsted procedure, named after a prominent breast surgeon from Johns Hopkins. This drastic breast cancer surgery, first performed by Dr. William Stewart Halsted in 1895, aims at removing the tumor, along with any surrounding tissues that may have become involved, including all major and minor pectoral muscles and all axillary lymph nodes. It demonstrated an initial understanding that cancer is a disease that spreads beyond what the naked eyes can see.

Through multiple randomized clinical trials, Dr. Bernard Fisher of the National Surgical Adjuvant Breast Project finally convinced many skeptical surgeons in the medical establishment that radical mastectomy is no better than simple mastectomy (breast removal without removing chest wall muscles). Moreover, Dr. Fisher showed that simple mastectomy is no better than breast conservation surgery through lumpectomy and adjuvant radiation.[6]

This is a big advance from Halsted's original procedure, since these newer approaches are much more patient-friendly and promote a better quality of life. For modern-day oncologists, these findings confirmed the observation that cancer is not just a locally invasive disease, but also a *systemic* disease requiring a systemic approach to control its spreading. Thus, the development of systemic chemotherapy to prevent the cancer from spreading, or metastasizing, had begun.

Dr. Gianni Bonadonna and his colleagues from Instituto Nazionale Tumori in Milan, Italy, conducted the first successful adjuvant breast cancer chemotherapy trial, using regimen CMF (cyclophosphamide, methotrexate, and fluorouracil) to reduce the risk of breast cancer recurrence after surgery. The preliminary results, published in 1975 and updated in 1981, showed that patients who received 85 percent of the total designated chemotherapy dosage had a five-year, relapse-free survival rate of 77 percent, while the comparable rate for patients who were treated only with a radical mastectomy was 45 percent.[7]

The CMF regimen therefore became the standard of care until the early 1990s, when another adjuvant chemotherapy protocol using a combination of adriamycin and cyclophosphamide was shown in multiple clinical trials to be either equivalent or slightly superior to the CMF regimen. The adriamycin/cyclophosphamide regimen then became the preferred adjuvant breast cancer treatment in the United States, although traditional CMF is still considered an effective and slightly safer choice for adjuvant breast cancer treatment.

In a twenty-year follow-up of the original 1995 study, Dr. Bonadonna published a report showing that patients in the treatment group receiving adjuvant combination chemotherapy had a 35 percent decrease in their rate of relapse, and that the risk of death dropped by 22 percent in all patient groups with positive node involvement except for postmenopausal women.

An interesting note concerning the evolution of the CMF regimen is that the original regimen used cyclophosphamide in small, daily, oral doses for fourteen days in a row during a twenty-eight-day treatment cycle. Later, a modified CMF regimen used cyclophosphamide at a much higher dose every three weeks. Multiple randomized clinical trials comparing modified high-dose CMF with traditional CMF showed that the high-dose regime was less effective than traditional CMF, which is now also called metronomic CMF.

A randomized clinical trial conducted by the Netherlands Cancer Institute demonstrated the superiority of the metronomic protocol for women with advanced breast cancer. The study found that classical or metronomic CMF induced a significant response rate of 48 percent versus 29 percent for the high-dose treatment, while the median survival rate for metronomic CMF was seventeen months versus twelve months for high-dose CMF.

The Netherlands Cancer Institute study may be one of the few randomized studies showing that giving a chemotherapy drug in smaller doses but more frequently might improve the efficacy of treatment. The improved efficacy of metronomic administration clearly demonstrates that the specific combination of chemotherapeutic drugs is not the only factor affecting treatment efficacy; dosing rate and treatment frequency also play a significant role.

All in all, these studies marked the first successes in using combination chemotherapy to effectively reduce the risk of cancer relapses after local and/or regional therapies. They also reaffirmed the understanding that cancer is a systemic disease that is often not curable by local therapies alone, including surgery and radiation treatments.

In the following years, numerous adjuvant studies in breast cancer and other tumor types such as colorectal cancer, gastroesophageal cancer, lung cancer, ovarian cancer, and pancreatic cancer, have established the roles of chemotherapy in combination with surgery and/or radiation as the standard of care in managing these cancers in their early stages.

THE "WAR ON CANCER"

During the late 1960s and into the 1970s, newly found successes in the treatment of acute leukemia, lymphomas, and breast cancer inspired the hope that cancer would soon be cured if more intensified research was instituted.

This led to the declaration of a "war on cancer" by President Richard Nixon with the passage of the National Cancer Act in 1971. By 2010, over $110 billion had been spent on cancer research. However, the war on cancer's goal of *curing* the disease has essentially failed.

From 1975 to 2006, cancer mortality rates have decreased slightly for men but not for women.[8] In men, the decrease is largely due to a decrease in smoking-related lung cancer deaths. For advanced malignancies that are not curable by complete surgical resection, only a handful of rare types of cancers, such as testicular cancer, choriocarcinoma, some lymphomas, and leukemia, which make up a small portion of all cancers, have proven to be curable. Most common solid tumors, once they reach an advanced stage, carry a poor prognosis with median survival rates ranging from a few months to a couple of years.

As the decades have worn on since the inception of the war on cancer, hope for treatment breakthroughs from progress in research has come and gone, not unlike fashion fads. An excellent illustration of a "cancer fad" was seen in 1998 when Dr. Judah Folkman of Harvard Medical School discovered two drugs that blocked tumors from generating new blood vessels in mice without causing any obvious side effects. This finding triggered such high optimism that the *New York Times* declared that a cancer cure was finally in sight. This hope was completely dashed several years later when these supposed wonder drugs failed to produce the same anticancer effects in human trials.[9]

The first drug targeting the specific biochemical changes caused by a specific type of cancer was developed in 2001. This targeted therapy was approved for the treatment of chronic myelogenous leukemia (CML). Like the previous successes of chemotherapy in certain rare cancers, the drug Gleevec proved to be a game-changer for the treatment of CML. Gleevec, along with several second- and third-generation drugs, have turned CML into an easily manageable and curable cancer. CML was once a truly dreadful disease, requiring high-dose chemotherapy with agents so toxic that bone marrow transplantation was required.

The development of targeted therapy ushered in a decade of efforts to find more of the same magic bullets for cancer, an approach described as "precision medicine." In his 2015 State of the Union address, President Obama described this effort as "a cancer treatment initiative."

The rapid advance in our ability to sequence human genomic DNA, coupled with computer-assisted drug development, increased the enthusiasm that many drugs would be found that would be effective on such difficult-to-treat cancers as lung cancer or melanoma. However, most human cancer DNA is so complex and variable that targeted therapy agents that are effective and long-lasting remain out of reach for most of the common cancers we face.

In the last couple of years, the central focus of the cancer community has been directed at the rediscovered treatment option of immunotherapy. This emphasis was triggered by the introduction of monoclonal antibodies to the PD-1 and PDL-1 checkpoint inhibitors. So far, these promising agents have induced durable remissions in small numbers of patients suffering from lung cancer, kidney cancer, bladder cancer, and melanoma.

Currently, the hope is very high that immunotherapy will lead to major improvements in cancer treatment outcomes. History has, however, frequently shown us that any single treatment modality, no matter how promising it may appear at first, is unlikely to make a qualitative difference in the overall management of cancer.

UNDERSTANDING CELLS

In order to understand the effects of any chemical agent or drug in the body, we must have a basic knowledge of cell structure and its relationship to our health. All cells form through the division of parent cells in a process called *mitosis*. The cell cycle can be divided into the following five phases:

> *Gap 0 phase*: This is the resting phase, when the cell is not dividing. The cell only comes out of this phase when it receives a signal to divide.
> *Gap 1 phase*: The cell enlarges and makes mRNA and proteins to ensure it is ready for the steps that lead to mitosis.
> *S or synthesis phase*: During this phase, DNA replication produces two new copies of DNA that can be passed onto the daughter cells produced by mitosis.
> *Gap 2 phase*: This phase is the period between the synthesis stage and the mitosis stage during which the cell continues to grow. A check-

point control mechanism ensures that the cell is ready to progress to mitosis.

M phase or mitosis: The cell no longer grows and begins dividing into two daughter cells. Another checkpoint mechanism ensures the cell is ready to divide.[10]

Cancer cells differ from normal cells in the way they grow and divide. When cells grow out of control, they may become cancerous and form new, abnormal cells, capable of invading other tissues and permeating the blood and lymphatic vessels that carry them to other sites in the body. This process of detachment, permeation, movement, and reestablishment is called *metastasis*, a property that normal cells do not possess.

CHEMOTHERAPY MECHANISMS FOR TARGETING CANCER CELLS

The main mechanism of chemotherapy agents is the disruption of the constant machinery of mitosis in cancer cells. Mitosis can be disrupted by inhibiting the synthesis of DNA, directly damaging the DNA of the cancer cell, or by inhibiting the proteins required for DNA replication and chromosome separation. These effects can directly kill the cancer cells, or induce the suicide of cancer cells called programmed cell death or *apoptosis*. Induction of apoptosis may be the most important pathway for chemotherapeutic agents, because some cancers that have high expression of an antiapoptotic protein called BCL-2 are, unsurprisingly, resistant to chemotherapy.

Since chemotherapy targets the proliferative mechanisms of cancer growth, cancers with large fractions of rapidly dividing cells, such as acute myelogenous leukemia and aggressive lymphomas, are typically more sensitive to antimitotic chemotherapy agents, and are good candidates for this type of treatment. However, fast-growing cancers may also develop new cellular or genomic mechanisms that render them resistant to cancer drugs that are initially effective. Moreover, some aggressive fast-growing cancers, such as malignant melanoma, may overgrow chemotherapy treatments and do not respond well to conventional chemotherapy in the first place.

In terms of the stages of mitosis affected, there are four basic classes of chemotherapeutic agents. Examples of the more common chemotherapeutic agents, the cell phases and functions they affect, and the cancers they treat most effectively, are as follows:

Alkylating agents—Alkylating agents damage DNA directly by permanently attaching a hydrocarbon fragment to one of the bases that comprises the backbone of the DNA molecule. These bonds prevent mitosis. Because alkylating agents affect the DNA molecule directly, they affect cancer cells at any phase of the cell cycle. Alkylating agents are used to treat leukemia, lymphomas, multiple myeloma, sarcoma and lung, breast, and ovarian cancers. Examples of drugs in this class include the following:

Nitrogen mustards: chlorambucil, cyclophosphamide, ifosfamide, and melphalan
Alkylsulfonates: busulfan
Nitrosoureas: streptozotocin, carmustine, and lomustine
Triazines: dacarbazine
Ethylenimines: thiotepa and altretamine
Platinum drugs: cisplatin, carboplatin, and oxaliplatin

Antimetabolites—Antimetabolites have similar structures to naturally occurring molecules used in the synthesis of biological molecules, like DNA or RNA. Although antimetabolites resemble chemicals needed for normal biochemical activity, they differ enough to interfere with normal cell function. These agents disrupt the S phase. They are used to treat leukemia and cancers of the gastrointestinal tract, breast, lung, and ovaries. Examples of drugs in this class include 5-fluorouracil (5-FU), 6-mercaptopurine (6-MP), cytarabine, capecitabine, fludarabine, gemcitabine, methotrexate, pemetrexed, pentostatin, and thioguanine.

Anthracyclines—Anthracyclines are antitumor antibiotics that inhibit the enzyme topoisomerase II that bring about DNA replication. They may also inhibit tumor DNA synthesis by causing oxidative DNA damage. Anthracyclines act at all phases of the cell cycle and are widely used for the treatments of many forms of cancer, including leukemia, lymphoma, sarcoma and breast cancer. Drugs in this class include doxorubicin, daunorubicin, idarubicin, and epirubicin.

Topoisomerase inhibitors—These agents inhibit the enzymes topoisomerase I and II, which would usually help untangle DNA strands so they can be replicated. They act during the Gap 2 phase and cause double strand DNA breaks. They are used to treat a broad spectrum of cancers including leukemia, lung, ovarian, and colon cancers and soft tissue sarcoma. Examples include topotecan, irinotecan as topoisomerase I inhibitors, adriamycin, etoposide, and teniposide as topoisomerase II inhibitors.

Plant alkaloids—Also called mitotic inhibitors, these drugs interrupt the M phase of the cell cycle and inhibit mitosis. They are used to treat many different cancers, such as breast and lung cancers, myeloma, lymphoma, and leukemia. Examples of drugs in this class include taxanes, such as paclitaxel and docetaxel, and vinca alkaloids, such as vinblastine, vincristine, and vinorelbine.

Corticosteroids—This drug class includes naturally occurring and artificially synthesized steroid hormones. They treat such cancers as lymphoma, leukemia, and multiple myeloma, and are used before chemotherapy to help prevent anaphylactic reactions, and after therapy to minimize nausea and vomiting. Examples include prednisone, methylprednisolone, and dexamethasone.[11]

Another important mechanism of cancer chemotherapy that has recently been proposed is called *chemo-induced immunogenic tumor cell death*. It is based on the finding that exposure to certain chemotherapy drugs can induce cancer cells to release a stress signal, such as the expression of intracellular proteins on the cell surface, or the alteration of the structure of the cell surface structure. These drug-induced changes serve as new antigens that stimulate the immune system to initiate an immune attack on the stressed cancer cells. A number of chemotherapy drugs have been found to have this capability, but usually when they are given at lower doses. We will examine the phenomenon of chemo-induced immunogenic tumor cell death in detail in chapter 3.

TREATMENT REGIMENS

Combination chemotherapy combines several drugs to exploit the synergy of different anticancer agents. Biologic agents that target certain specific cancer growth mechanisms that are not directly related to cell proliferation are often included in the combination to enhance the effects of traditional chemotherapy agents. For example, bevacizumab, a monoclonal antibody against tumor vascular endothelia growth factor (VEGF), is usually added to combination chemotherapy for lung, colon, and brain cancers.

Combining drugs in a chemotherapy regimen is typically more effective than single agent chemotherapy. Combination chemotherapy has led to cures in such chemo-sensitive cancers as choriocarcinoma, testicular cancers, and malignant lymphomas, even in their advanced stages. However, combination chemotherapy also tends to have more side effects, especially when all drugs are given at maximally tolerated doses.

Concurrent chemoradiotherapy refers to a combination of radiotherapy and chemotherapy drug(s) chosen to enhance the effectiveness of the radiation. This is often done when radiation is given with curative intent for certain types of intermediate stage cancers, such as head and neck cancer, lung cancer, and bladder cancer. Although it is generally well tolerated, side effects from both treatment modalities can be significant.

Neoadjuvant and *adjuvant chemotherapy* refer to chemotherapy given in association with surgery. Neoadjuvant chemotherapy refers to the administration of chemotherapy prior to surgery in an effort to shrink tumors to a size small enough for resection. Adjuvant chemotherapy refers to chemotherapy given after surgical removal of a tumor to reduce the risk of relapse. The duration and extent of these treatments are usually determined by clinical trials in which the effectiveness of various doses and durations are determined.

In practice, patients are usually infused with drugs at intervals ranging from every week to every three or four weeks under the supervision of hospital or cancer clinic physicians. The treatment course typically lasts an average of three to six months for adjuvant chemotherapy, but may be of indefinite length when treating stage 4 cancers so long as the cancer remains under control and the patient continues to tolerate the treatment.

It is, however, important to recognize that almost all treatment regimens suffer from one significant weakness. Most regimens include a built-in break between treatment cycles during which the patient recovers from the side effects of treatment. Unfortunately, this break may provide a respite for the cancer cells under attack, allowing them to recover and sometimes even develop a resistance to further treatment. Moreover, it has been shown that the likelihood of cancer recovery *increases with the duration of the break*.

The issue of cancer recovery/resistance will be discussed in chapter 3. One of the major issues that will be discussed there is the way in which metronomic low-dose chemotherapy can be used to prevent the development of resistance in cancer cells.

SIDE EFFECTS OF CHEMOTHERAPY

Because cancer cells usually grow and divide more rapidly than normal cells, chemotherapy can selectively kill cancer cells while affecting normal cells to a much lesser extent. However, some normal cells, such as bone marrow cells, epithelial cells lining the digestive tract (mouth, stomach, intestines, esophagus), as well as the reproductive system and hair follicles cells, do multiply relatively fast, and chemotherapy can affect them as well.

Chemotherapy causes side effects such as low blood cell counts, fatigue, nausea and vomiting, diarrhea, and hair loss. Chemotherapy may occasionally affect cells of vital organs, such as the heart, kidney, bladder, lungs, and nervous system.

As doctors in the final two decades of the last century began taking an aggressive approach in treating cancer with drug regimens, this meant their patients were also facing a continual struggle with harsh side effects. Fortunately, the last decade has witnessed the development of much more satisfying supportive agents for cancer chemotherapy, including the availability of multiple effective short- and long-acting antinausea medications, and the development of several bone marrow growth factors that can increase the production of red and white blood cells following chemotherapy. In general, the awareness of unusual but severe side effects from some chemotherapy agents and closer monitoring protocols has made chemotherapy safer.

While the supportive care agents have made high-dose chemotherapy generally tolerable, some side effects are more disguised. One of the most serious disguised side effects of high-dose chemotherapy is its adverse impact on the immune system. Indeed, the chemotherapy-induced suppression of the immune system may be the main reason conventional chemotherapy so often fails.

THE BOTTLENECK OF CONVENTIONAL CHEMOTHERAPY

Although the use of chemotherapy saw initial success in the treatment of several chemo-sensitive cancers, it has had limited success against most solid tumors in advanced stages. After administering conventional chemotherapy, the improvement in survival rates for patients with stage 4 cancers usually ranges from a few weeks to a few months. Over the years, much effort and many resources have been spent on clinical trials intended to evaluate different drug combinations and cancer protocols. All too often no significant difference has been found between experimental and comparison treatments. For example, after initial finding that chemotherapy improved the longevity and quality of life of stage 4 lung cancer patients, very little subsequent progress has been seen; the median survival rate of such patients has ranged from ten months to several years, regardless of the combination of chemotherapy drugs administered. This stagnation is a clear sign that the current research methodology of randomized trials among different chemotherapy combinations has reached its limit.

The poor results of treating patients with advanced solid tumors with conventional chemotherapy have spawned pessimism in the medical community. This perception of futility has led some physicians to refer patients with advanced cancers to hospice prematurely. Indeed, traditional chemotherapy effects on most common solid tumors may have hit a wall despite development of increasing numbers of new drugs.

The lack of enough research on the best ways to give chemotherapy agents, in particular regarding the dosages and frequency of administration is at least partly to blame for this stagnation in the improvement of chemotherapy effectiveness. The principle of current chemotherapy treatment is still dominated by the decades-old "log-kill" theory of tumor cells, which declares that each chemotherapy dose kills a defined log fraction of tumor cells, hence the higher the dose of chemo drugs, the more cancer cells they can kill. This theory was developed from leukemia disease models and does not apply well to solid tumors from organs like lung and breasts. Nonetheless, the log-kill model has led to the doctrine of maximum tolerated dose (MTD) chemotherapy for all cancer treatment. This may be directly responsible for the lack of efficacy of chemotherapy for solid tumors, with many caveats including high treatment toxicity, immunosuppression, and tumor resistance (see chapter 4 for more discussions on this subject in relation to metronomic chemotherapy). Throughout this book I will discuss how, by changing the rhythm (dose and frequency) of the chemotherapy administration, we can make a big difference in its efficacy for most common solid tumors. We have seen numerous patients who have been told to "put their affairs in order," only to survive for many years after a fundamental change in their treatment plan.

To improve cancer treatment outcomes, we need new, truly innovative thinking.

The recent development of targeted therapies and immunotherapies has compounded the problems associated with improving the efficacy of chemotherapy. The promise of these newer approaches has pushed chemotherapy into the background of ongoing research efforts. This diminution of effort is unfortunate, because chemotherapy not only is still the dominant treatment modality relied on by most cancer patients, it actually has certain advantages when compared to targeted therapies.

For example, chemotherapy is still more effective in treating most cancers that don't carry specific, targetable mutations. It is estimated that the DNA of many cancers have more than five hundred different genetic mutations. This abundance often makes it impossible to determine which specific mutation is a major driver of cancer growth, or how changing any given mutation will change the behavior of other related mutations.

The fact that many alternative mutations can control cancer means that treatments targeting a specific mutation often result in the development of resistance. With a few exceptions, this approach is also unlikely to lead to major tumor destruction; the high genetic heterogeneity found in advanced cancers makes it quite likely that a treatment targeting a specific mutation will miss one or more genetic subtypes and select for resistant cancer cell clones. Conversely, chemotherapy kills cancer cells because it targets the biochemical processes driving rapid proliferation, and these processes are similar in all kinds of cancers. Moreover, if chemotherapy is given at the right dose, it can kill cancer cells without having a major impact on normal cells or the immune system. For these and other reasons, it is imperative that more studies be conducted on new and better ways of administering chemotherapy. Specifically, studies are needed on using low-dose chemotherapy as a foundation for other new therapies, including targeted therapy and immunotherapy.

In summary, chemotherapy affects rapid cell division, which is potentially the most effective method we have in fighting cancer. If administered correctly, by using the protocol of metronomic low-dose chemotherapy (chapter 3), it can be a powerful weapon. This potential is significantly increased if metronomic low-dose chemotherapy is used in a synergistic combination with the innovative and integrative methods under development today. The potential of combined therapies is discussed in chapters 5 and 6.

THE FUTURE OF TRADITIONAL CHEMOTHERAPY

We have now come to see that chemotherapy is an important weapon in our anti-cancer arsenal. Chemotherapy can also be the foundation of future cancer treatment paradigms involving targeted therapy and immunotherapy. On the other hand, existing chemotherapy methodology hampered by the doctrine of maximum tolerated dose administration clearly has vast room for improvement because of its lack of consistent efficacy, well-known toxicity, and immunosuppressive effects.

In addition to changing the dosing and tempo of the chemotherapy drugs given as discussed above, a very promising method of enhancing the precision and hence the effectiveness of chemotherapy is the use of chemotherapy "smart bombs": a delivery system that greatly increases the proportion of drug molecules that actually enters cancer cells. One such approach to precision targeting is linking a chemotherapy drug to a monoclonal antibody that targets an antigen on the surface of cancer cells. Such an approach brings the chemotherapy molecule into direct physical contact with cancer cells. When the monoclonal antibody bonds to the surface antigen, the drug is brought inside the cancer cells by a process called *endocytosis*.

An example of a drug of this type that is currently on the market is Kadcyla, which is generally used on a specific type of breast cancer overproducing the growth-stimulating protein receptors called HER2-Neu on the cell surface. This makes breast cancer cells grow and divide in an uncontrolled way. Trastuzumab (Herceptin) is a monoclonal antibody that attaches itself to the HER2 protein. Kadcyla is a combination of Herceptin and the chemotherapy drug emtansine by a chemical link. Kadcyla therefore delivers emtansine directly to cancer cells when trastuzumab attaches to HER2 protein. Kadcyla is both effective and generally well tolerated.

Another way to deliver cancer drugs more precisely to their targets is to package them into nanoparticles that can be more specifically picked up by cancer cells. Depending on their size, nanoparticles can penetrate tumor tissues more easily than the drug by itself. The time nanoparticle drugs are retained in cancerous cells is also longer than for drugs that are not packaged into nanoparticles.

The surface features of the nanoparticle facilitate entry into cancer cells by a process called *ligand-receptor interaction*. An example of such a drug delivery approach is the chemotherapy drug called albumin-bound paclitaxel (Abraxane). This chemotherapy drug is currently approved for treating several different cancers, including breast, ovarian, lung, and pancreatic cancers. It consists of a generic drug called paclitaxel, which is packaged into albumin-coated nanoparticles. It is believed that cancer cells pick up the albumin nanoparticles by *transcytosis*, which is facilitated by albumin receptors on the surface of the cancer cell.

Kadcyla and Abraxane represent two of the earlier models of targeted chemotherapy drug delivery. The next decade will likely see more delivery methods like this, which will increase the efficacy of chemotherapy.

Improved supportive care may also significantly improve the efficacy of chemotherapy. The development of more effective antiemetics and marrow supportive growth factors over the last decade has already made chemotherapy safer and more tolerable. More supportive care measures, such as pharmaceutical interventions, and integrative treatments, such as exercises, nutrition, and mind-body medicine, may combine to improve the quality of life and even the treatment outcomes for patients undergoing chemotherapy.

A MOST CRUCIAL EQUATION

We know that chemotherapy inadvertently took wing after a series of accidents, leading scientists to believe that toxic chemicals can kill cancerous cells and lead to a cure. Initially, it was believed that more was better; that giving these drugs at doses as high as the patient could tolerate would achieve the best results.

However, decades of this practice have shown it reflects an erroneous belief. In the case of chemotherapy, it seems to be true that *less is more*. A reaction against the MTD mind-set may have originally motivated some scientists from Harvard University to begin experimenting with giving chemotherapy drugs at lower doses, but more frequently. One of their initial findings was that this process greatly reduced the incidence of the development of drug-resistant cancers. Another finding was that the enhanced efficacy of metronomic low-dose chemotherapy depended on the competence of the patient's immune system, which clearly indicates that this treatment modality works *through the immune system* to control the cancer.

Unfortunately, these important preclinical studies of metronomic low-dose chemotherapy did not gain much traction in clinical practice because of the fixation of the entire oncology community on using MTD treatments. Ironically, the only segment of the medical community who paid attention to these early studies was the veterinarian community. Veterinarians began to integrate metronomic low-dose chemotherapy into their practice of treating animals with cancer, a practice that has become commonplace today.

The idea of using chemotherapy in tandem with the immune system to control cancer is intuitively appealing. A corollary of such a belief is the importance of maintaining a balance between killing cancer cells and maintaining a competent immune system that can recognize and control the cancer in the long run. This is a crucial equation, one that invites an integrative approach to cancer treatment—killing the cancer while simultaneously boosting the immune system.

Before exploring why less is more, as we will do in chapter 3, it is important to understand the importance of a healthy immune system. This is your key to good health, from preventing a simple cold to surviving cancer. We will provide an overview of the function of the immune system in the following chapter.

2

IN DEFENSE OF OUR HEALTH

The Role of the Immune System
in Cancer Prevention and Control

When you first see Darrel, he just appears to be a very healthy-looking eighty-three-year-old man. Then, upon looking more closely, you notice a urinary bag strapped to his leg like the holster of a gun. That's because Darrel is a survivor of invasive bladder cancer diagnosed fifteen years ago. It had developed from an early-stage bladder cancer for which he was being monitored and treated by a urologist. Since the cancer then had penetrated the muscle wall of his bladder, he received concurrent chemo-radiation with low-dose chemotherapy and the cancer appeared to have gone away in a follow-up cystoscopy. However, the cancer grew back in the bladder and beyond its wall about a year later, and this time his urologist performed a drastic surgery to remove the bladder entirely, leaving him with the urinary bag. Just as he was recovering from the surgery, the cancer recurred and progressed again to the rim of his pelvis and several lymph nodes in his groin area. A biopsy revealed that it was the same bladder cancer, but by then it had become a full-blown stage 4 disease. Darrel was treated with weekly metronomic low-dose chemo-therapy consisting of gemcitabine, paclitaxel, and carboplatin, along with a gamut of supplements to stimulate his immune system. Miraculously, his cancer went away again. This time, he was placed on a protocol of low-dose interferon injected into his skin three times a week, a regimen that regularly provides his immune system with the boost it needs. Over the past thirteen years, this treatment, along with a collection of supplements he continually takes, became part of Darrel's life routine. Follow-up PET-CT scans over the years continued to light up several lymph nodes deep in his abdomen, which remained suspicious for active residual cancer, but Darrel and the cancer seem to have established a truce. Without any further treatment, no new or spreading cancer has ever been found again. Other than a small bout of mini-strokes (transient ischemic attacks or TIAs) a few years ago, Darrel's life has mostly been healthy, even vibrant.

Darrel's case is proof that cancer, even at its advanced stages, can be turned into a chronic disease that we can coexist with. This stalemate between cancer and the body's immune system that controls it is called *immune equilibrium* (see later). Darrel's initial treatment consisted of low-dose chemotherapy that helped preserve and ignited the inner immune system response against his cancer, which was further maintained with integrative therapies as well as immunotherapies. Of note, in the first two years of his long cancer journey, he had two relapses or progressions of his cancer. Both times cancer was beaten back with the same treatment and was followed with the same maintenance therapies. The perseverance paid off. After five years from his initial diagnosis, Darrel's cancer never flared up again. It's like a seesaw war that was lastly won by Darrel's immune system.

WHAT IS THE IMMUNE SYSTEM?

The immune system is a vital caretaker that protects us from such foreign invaders as bacteria, viruses, fungi, the toxic chemicals produced by microbes. Mounting evidence also shows that the immune system plays an important role in preventing the development of cancer and continues to play a role in limiting its growth after it has developed. To reiterate, the health of the immune system may be the single most important factor in determining our survival after a cancer diagnosis.

THE STRUCTURES AND FUNCTIONS OF THE IMMUNE SYSTEM

Our immune system consists of the different organs, cells, and proteins that work together to fight the harmful effects of foreign organisms and toxins as well as cancer. Immunologists divide the immune system into two parts, based on how they react to new antigens—the innate and adaptive immune system.

The *innate immune system* is evolutionarily ancient, found in various degrees from single-celled organisms to humans. We are born with it, and from the beginning it is ready to fight foreign intruders, including cancer, without any need of prior activation. It is our front-line defense against these diseases. When an infection or cancer is not cleared by this innate system, it can usher in the second phase of the immune attack from the *adaptive immune system*, which we will discuss soon.

The innate immune system starts with the skin and membranous tissues lining our organs as barriers to foreign intruders or invading cancer cells. This barrier system includes various types of immune cells, some of which are particularly important in fighting cancer. One of the most important innate immune system cells are called *natural killer* (NK) cells. These cells express unique receptors, called NKG2D, that can engage the NKG2D ligands present on tumor cells—but not on normal cells—and initiate specific immune attacks to destroy the tumor cells.[1] Activated NK cells also produce cytokines that further enhances the immune reaction and activated secondary immune responses. Another vital cellular part of the innate immune system is the *phagocyte*, which can basically engulf tumor cells or collect their debris after they are destroyed. An especially important type of phagocyte, the *dendritic cell*, processes engulfed tumor cells and embeds pieces of the tumor in peptide form on its surface. Dendritic cells then present these peptide fragments to immune effector cells, including T and B cells, and activate them. These activated immune effector cells then expand in numbers and can eliminate tumor cells bearing the same antigen as the one presented on the dendritic cells. The cytokine immune mediators produced during the immune response then initiate a cascade of secondary, or "adaptive," immune responses directed against the tumor cells, eventually leading to their destruction.

Cancer cells can generate telltale antigens through the very perturbations that render them malignant, in response to the cellular "stress" from the abnormal cell proliferation and the subsequent inflammation it causes.[2] For instance, viral transformation of normal cells into malignant cells can also stimulate the cancer cells to produce NKG2D ligands, to which the NK cells can bind. This binding activates NK cells, which then engulf the tumor cells and break down their membranes through a process called *lysis*. In doing so, the NK cell produces other immune response mediators that augment subsequent adaptive immune responses.

The adaptive immune system is the part of the immune system that responds more specifically to certain parts of the cancer or foreign cells. It consists of *lymphocytes* (T and B lymphocytes) that bear receptors that recognize unique structures on the surface of the cancer cells. Unlike NK cells, T cells need to be activated first through interaction with antigen-presenting cells in the body, such as dendritic cells. Once activated, they can start attacking the antigen-bearing cancer cells through an interaction between T-cell receptors and tumor antigens.[3]

Initially, T cells bear such a wide variety of tumor antigen receptors that their effectiveness against any particular antigen/tumor type is not very great. However, the immune response is also a self-propagating process that is augmented by *cytokines*, *interleukins*, and *interferons*, which are produced by activating immune cells themselves.

The immune response can become stronger as more tumors are destroyed, which in turn stimulates further immune response. Unlike the innate immune system, the adaptive immune system stores memories of what has happened. When the intrusive antigen from microorganisms or cancer are detected a second time, the adaptive immune system mounts a much swifter and stronger response to clear these antigens.

Cancer cells always mutate due to their genetic instability. The adaptive immune system, being a product of human evolution, has a built-in ability to adapt its responses to millions of antigens. Theoretically, it can also adapt to the constant changes of cancer cells much more effectively and rapidly than we can develop drugs in a laboratory.

Because of this innate ability of the immune system to fight the cancer, it is very important to maintain the vitality of our immune system during cancer treatment.

THE THEORY OF CANCER IMMUNE EDITING

It has long been suspected that the immune system plays a surveillance role in the development of cancer by first identifying cells that carry mutation-induced structural alterations and then eliminating them. We have seen evidence of this in the animal models that carry inherent defects in key innate immune system components, such as NK cells. These animals almost invariably develop cancer. It has also been discovered that cancer can sometimes reach a state of equilibrium with active immune responses such that it can for a time remain stable in size and location. Usually, however, these stalemated tumors may eventually develop mutations that allow them to evade the immune system completely, at least so long as the microenvironment remains the same.

The three phases of interaction between the immune system and cancer—immune surveillance, immune equilibrium, and immune evasion—are called cancer *immune editing*. This theory lays the foundation for our current understanding of the interaction between the immune system and cancer, and provides guidance for our strategies in optimizing the immune system to prevent the development of cancer, to treat the cancer, and to reduce the risk of its recurrence.[4]

IMMUNE SURVEILLANCE

In 1909, Paul Ehrlich initially proposed the influence of the immune system in preventing the development of cancer when he suggested that the immune system repressed cancer development, which would otherwise occur at a high frequency. Half a century later, in 1957, Burnett and Thomas formulated the concept of cancer immune surveillance. However, the validation of this concept did not occur until the early 1990s when technical developments in the world of molecular biology enabled researchers to specifically knock out genes encoding components of the immune system, making it possible to evaluate the roles of these immune components in the development of cancer.[5] These studies not only demonstrated the presence of immune surveillance of cancer, it also implied the importance of intact immune system components and functions in carrying out this process for an organism's survival.

The initial studies involved knocking out the important immune mediator *interferon gamma* and the *perforins*. The animals that had these modulators knocked out had an enhanced susceptibility to both chemically induced and spontaneous tumor generation. This finding strongly suggested the action of immune mediators in preventing tumor development. Another study employed gene-targeted mice lacking the recombinant-activating gene RAG–2, which demonstrated that lymphocytes expressing rearranged antigen receptors played critical roles in the cancer immune surveillance process. In one study, thirty-one of thirty-two RAG-2 mutant mice developed spontaneous tumors, whereas only twelve out of thirty-three wild mice developed tumors by the end of their lives.

The importance of NK cells in immune surveillance was directly demonstrated by depletion of NK cells with monoclonal antibodies to the NK 1.1 antigen. Mice that lacked NK cells were two to three times more susceptible to carcinogen-induced cancer development. It was later demonstrated that NK cells, through binding with receptors NKG2D to tumor-specific ligands such as MIC A/B proteins, can initiate automatic tumor destruction. It has been further demonstrated that inflammation associated with tumor development can upregulate tumor-specific antigens, such as MIC A/B proteins, leading to NK cell activation.[6]

An eleven-year follow-up study of 154 healthy individuals also found that individuals with high to medium-high NK cell activity in their peripheral bloodstream had a 40 percent lower risk of developing cancer than those with low NK cell activity.[7]

A related study found that individuals with a high incidence of familial cancers had a much lower NK cell count than people with no significant familial history of cancers, again suggesting that defects in natural NK cell activity may play a role in the initial stages of human tumorigenesis. This finding indicates that it may be possible to identify individuals at increased risk of cancer by measuring NK cell activity.[8]

Taken together, these studies have confirmed the importance of both the innate and the adaptive immune system in preventing cancer development. To reduce the risk of cancer relapse or recurrences, we must not damage the immune system and also keep it healthy throughout the cancer treatment.

IMMUNE EQUILIBRIUM

The clinical scenario that most clearly demonstrates the existence of the equilibrium phase of the immune tumor interaction occurs when an organ from a host with a long history of cancer is transplanted into an immuno-compromised recipient taking immunosuppressive medicines to prevent organ rejection. Although the organ donor in these studies had been cancer free for many years, the recipient soon developed the same type of tumor that had previously existed in the donor. The equilibrium that the donor cancer cells had reached with the donor immune system was lost in the immunocompromised transplant recipient.

Although the equilibrium phase of a tumor/immune system interaction is not completely understood, there are three possible outcomes for tumor cells that enter the latent period of equilibrium:

1. Eventual elimination by the immune system
2. Permanent maintenance of equilibrium
3. Escape from the immune control

Immune equilibrium refers to that state in which a cancer patient has been in stable condition or in a state of remission following anticancer treatment. The longer this phase lasts, the longer the patient will enjoy a period in which the cancer does not progress without additional intervention. To prolong the immune equilibrium phase is to minimize cancer activity while cultivating strong anticancer immune responses.[9] Since cancer cells typically develop apoptosis when they cannot grow or proliferate, it's possible that after a long equilibrium, cancer cells can be permanently eliminated by the immune system.

It is important to note that high-dose cancer chemotherapy, the dominant approach in today's traditional cancer centers, actually *weakens* the immune system, and likely contributes to the shortened periods of remission following treatment seen in many patients with advanced stage cancers.

IMMUNE EVASION

Eventually, the tumor usually escapes immune suppression. At this stage, the early surveillance mechanisms of the immune system have failed and cancer starts to grow again.

Multiple mechanisms may allow a tumor to escape from immune suppression. These mechanisms may include loss of tumor antigens, a loss of response to such immune mediators as interferon gamma, production of immunosuppressive cytokines, such as TGF-beta, or the development of immunosuppressive cells, such as *T regulatory cells* (Treg cells) and *myeloid derived suppressor cells* (MDSC).

A breakdown of the body's immune system also occurs when it is depleted of key nutrients essential for its proper function, or when external toxins suppress the immune system cells.[10]

It has been found that continuous tumor development can induce active Treg cells that suppress immune reaction against cancers by CD8 cytotoxic T cells and NK cells. Increased Treg cell activity occurring between chemotherapy cycles may thus allow tumor regrowth, reducing the efficacy of conventional chemotherapy. Therefore, cancer cannot be treated successfully by simply stimulating the immune system; *measures must also be taken to circumvent immunosuppression.*

It is important to note that metronomic low-dose chemotherapy can down-regulate Treg cells and MDSC cells, thereby enhancing the anti-tumor immune reaction.

Other mechanisms that enable cancer to evade the immune system include induction of T-cell apoptosis through PD-1/PDL-1 interaction, induction of inflammation, which in turn suppresses positive immune responses to cancer, and development of malnutrition during cancer treatment, which also can weaken any immune system function.

THE CORRELATION OF IMMUNE SYSTEM FUNCTION TO CANCER TREATMENT OUTCOMES

Despite the ability of tumors to evade the immune system during its development, the immune system still plays a vital role in limiting the growth and metastasis of tumors. It is the most important factor in determining any cancer treatment outcome. In general, we can predict that anticancer treatment will be more successful if there is a strong preexisting, antitumor immune response.

One important preexisting antitumor response is the level of circulating NK cell activity. It's been found in the case of uterine and colorectal cancers that low blood NK cell activity is associated with increased risk of metastasis. Although most human tumors are very resistant to infiltration by NK cells, the cancers that do allow significant NK cell infiltration, such as colorectal, lung, renal, gastric, and vulvar cancers, respond to NK cell infiltration with an improved prognosis and a reduction in tumor recurrence.

The extent of NK cell infiltration of peritumoral tissue (tissue surrounding a tumor) can also predict the likelihood of achieving a good pathological response or pathological complete response following neoadjuvant chemotherapy.[11]

In a study published in *Journal of Translational Medicine* in 2015 by Verma et al., patients with large, locally advanced breast cancers were generally found to have much less NK cell activity in their blood compared to normal individuals. Conversely, those who had higher levels of peritumoral NK cell infiltration had a much better chance of achieving a good to complete pathological response to neoadjuvant chemotherapy.[12]

Over the last few years, monoclonal antibodies have been developed that disrupt the suppressive effect of PD-1 and PDL-1 interactions on immune T cells. This disruption, which leads to T-cell activation and cancer control, has stirred strong interest in the field of cancer immunotherapy. The success of this treatment indicates that the immune system can still fight cancer despite the occurrence of an initial tumor escape—that is, if we can find a way to release its power. It's been found that the success of the anti-PD1/PDL-1 immunotherapy depends on the degree of tumor infiltration by immune T cells before treatment. If a tumor is not already infiltrated by immune cells, it is called a "cold tumor," and it does not respond well to immunotherapy. On the contrary, if a tumor is highly infiltrated by immune cells before immunotherapy, it is called a "hot tumor," and it likely would respond to immunotherapy well. This indicates a baseline immune system function is important for any cancer treatment including immunotherapy to work.

Unlike what we would like to believe, there is no single treatment that can activate the immune system and wipe out the existence of cancer. Instead, a comprehensive, integrative approach, including metronomic low-dose chemotherapy, diet, nutrition, exercise, mind-body therapy, and pharmaceutical intervention is more likely to lead to a successful treatment.

WHAT WE CAN LEARN FROM OUR PATIENTS

Merle had been working as an airline mechanic for almost thirty years when he started experiencing increasing nasal sinus congestion, along with headaches, and left facial numbness just over three years ago. Initially, Merle thought it was just another bout of sinusitis that had come and gone over the past five years. However, this time the symptoms kept getting worse, and he asked his primary care physician to refer him to an ear, nose, and throat (ENT) doctor. The nasal sinus endoscopic examination conducted by the specialist even surprised the doctor. Merle's two left paranasal sinuses were filled up with abnormal tissues, which were producing a swamp of thick mucus.

An MRI of Merle's head and sinuses brought more bad news. The sinuses around his nose were full of cancerous tissue, which had also extended to the base of his skull and the space behind his left eye, threatening to invade both the eye and the brain.

A biopsy from Merle's sinus tissue came back showing adenoid cystic carcinoma, a rare cancer usually found in the salivary gland under the mandibles. It's even more rare to find it in the sinuses. Merle was initially referred to a major teaching hospital and saw another well-known ENT surgeon, who determined that Merle's cancer was not operable due to the extent of its tissue involvement.

Merle was referred to medical and radiation oncology, but the only option he was given was palliative radiation for the area containing the most critical tumor located in the retroorbital space at the base of the skull. The radiation oncologist was very blunt in telling Merle that soon after the treatment began, the radiation would almost surely cause brain injury and blindness in the left eye, due to the close proximity of the tumors to these fragile areas.

After seeking a second opinion from me, Merle began receiving metronomic low-dose chemotherapy, along with cetuximab, a drug that targets the tumor cells while attracting the immune cells to the tumor site. After three months of this treatment, Merle's tumor had shrunk by 25 percent. After another three months, the tumor did not shrink or grow. From there, we placed him on a regimen of maintenance with cetuximab. He did fairly well, with minimal symptoms, and MRI scans administered every three months showed that the tumor was stable. This equilibrium lasted for some time, but eventually broke down. Merle developed more headaches and started to have very blurred vision in his left eye and trouble moving his left eye to the left lateral corner. An additional MRI showed a slight increase in the size of the tumor behind Merle's left eye and in the sinus around his nose.

At that time, a new immunotherapy drug called pambrolizumab (Keytruda) had been approved for treating head and neck squamous cell cancer that had progressed after chemotherapy. So we started Merle on this treatment. Three months later, Merle seemed to enter another state of equilibrium; his symptoms neither worsened nor improved.

Considering that metronomic low-dose chemotherapy can potentially enhance antitumor immune response, Merle was started on concurrent chemotherapy with the immunotherapy. His symptoms soon started to improve with decreasing left facial numbness and improving left eye vision.

At his next ENT checkup—and for the first time in three years—Merle's ENT doctor told him that the tumors in his sinuses were subsiding.

Merle's case illustrates the entire cancer immune editing process, from the prolonged latency phase of tumor development, to immune equilibrium achieved after receiving treatment, to tumor progression with immune evasion, and the return to immune equilibrium after combined therapy with immune-enhancing therapeutics and metronomic low-dose chemotherapy.

It's also an example of how the interaction between the immune system and cancer is a dynamic process and not a one-way street. That's because cancer can break through immune surveillance after evading the immune system. However, with the correct interventions, the equilibrium between cancer and the immune system can be reestablished. These processes may be repeated many times before a prolonged truce or immune equilibrium can finally be established.

THE EFFECTS OF HIGH-DOSE CHEMOTHERAPY ON THE IMMUNE SYSTEM

Studies have found that high-dose chemotherapy can induce a long-lasting immunosuppression that facilitates a recurrence of cancer. For example, a study found that conventional high-dose chemotherapy given in an adjuvant setting to a breast cancer patient after surgery caused an immunosuppressive effect on various immune effector cells that can last for months to over a year.[13]

MTD chemotherapy can also increase the numbers and activities of MDSC and Treg cells, leading to further immunosuppression. A study points to the role of activated Treg cells in the recovery of cancer cells between chemotherapy cycles and the eventual development of resistance to the chemotherapy treatment. Interestingly, MDSC cells have been found to "capture" blood circulating T cells, thereby preventing them from entering tissues and lymph nodes, which has the effect of disabling these important tumor-fighting immune cells.

Levels of malnutrition related to decreased appetite, nausea, vomiting, and diarrhea—all caused by high-dose chemotherapy—also contribute to immune suppression. There is increasing evidence that certain micronutrients, such as zinc, selenium, iron, copper, folic acid, and vitamins A, B6, C, and E are also important in maintaining normal immune cell functions. Cancer patients who have difficulty maintaining a regular and variable diet are prone to developing a deficiency of these micronutrients, along with an associated immunodeficiency.

In light of the immunosuppressive impact of MTD chemotherapy and the importance of the immune system to controlling cancer, it shouldn't be surprising that MTD chemotherapy often induces only a short-term tumor response, followed by the development of tumor resistance and a more aggressive phase of the disease.

Attention must be paid not only to the initial efficacy of a regimen of chemotherapy, but to the impact the treatment has on a person's immune system.

It is also imperative that the immune response be proactively strengthened at the same time as chemotherapy is being administered. Some researchers argue that a general stimulation of the immune system can be counterproductive, and that only the effector arm of the immune system, the part that attacks foreign invaders and tumors, should be stimulated. More specifically, some oncologists worry that a general strengthening of the immune system might entail a strengthening of the regulatory arm of the system, which might suppress the activity of effector cells and neutralize their anticancer benefits.

This shortsighted view of the immune system probably stems from a systemic bias against complementary and alternative medicine. While it is probably true that general immune supportive measures do not distinguish between regulatory versus effector arms, it is still important to keep the whole immune system healthy to maximize the favorable impacts of any type of intervention.

Cures and remissions are ultimately attributable to a robust immune system and, in turn, the vitality of the immune system is dependent on a healthy microenvironment. Indeed, without a healthy microenvironment, there may be no immune response at all. As has been shown in this chapter, a cancer patient without a competent immune system will derive only minimal benefits from anticancer treatments. In this respect they are very like AIDS patients, whose minor infection sometimes cannot be controlled even by powerful antibiotics due to defect in the basic immune system function.

Metronomic low-dose chemotherapy has repeatedly been shown to have the ability to modulate the immune system to enhance its response to tumors. This contrasts with conventional high-dose chemotherapy, which consistently suppresses the immune system in general. The immunosuppressive impact of MTD therapy will be discussed in detail in the next chapter.

MORE LESSONS FROM OUR PATIENTS

Richard is a sixty-five-year-old U.S. Army veteran who became suddenly ill about six years ago with intermittent abdominal pain associated with vomiting blood and having dark-reddish blood in his frequent bowel movements. At the emergency room, he was found to be dangerously anemic and received four pints of blood. Emergent upper endoscopy found cauliflower-like tumorous tissue in his duodenum. Biopsy showed a cancer called "poorly differentiated carcinoma with partial squamous differentiation." CT scan showed a large tumor mass of over 8cm was present in the triangular area formed by the duodenum, liver, and gallbladder, with apparent invasion of liver itself. A well-known liver surgeon saw him and decided that the tumor was not operable due to its size and multiorgan involvement. He was recommended conventional chemotherapy. He heard about me through a friend and came to see me as soon as he got out of hospital. After consultation, I immediately started him on a combination metronomic chemotherapy that we have successfully used for several types of gastrointestinal malignancy, consisting of paclitaxel, oxaliplatin, leucovorin, and 5-FU. Within a week, he felt his abdominal pain had eased up and bleeding decreased. After two more weeks, his bleeding stopped completely. After three months of treatment, a repeat CT scan showed the tumor had shrunk by more than 50 percent. Richard was referred to another surgeon and was deemed operable this time. Surgery was successful with en-bloc removal of the residual tumor and attached duodenum, gallbladder, and a portion of his liver. The pathology showed the tumor was most consistent with a metastatic gallbladder cancer. Since there was cancer left on the surgical margin, he received further radiation therapy to the surgical bed with concurrent low-dose chemotherapy. After nearly a year, Richard's cancer was finally in remission. He was started on a combination immune-boosting supplements and low-dose interferon, which he religiously followed for the next five years. He had completely regained his health and more. To this date, over six years after his initial diagnosis of an aggressive stage 4 cancer invading the liver, he has stayed in complete remission with better health than before he became sick. This is another example that even with advanced aggressive cancer, complete recovery and return to long-lasting immune equilibrium is possible if we treat the cancer with immune-enhancing metronomic low-dose chemo and support the immune system with integrative therapies at the same time.

HOW CAN WE ENHANCE OUR IMMUNE SYSTEM TO RESIST CANCER?

It is important to realize that cancers that can be detected by conventional imaging have already evaded immune system surveillance and broken out of immune equilibrium. Thus, in a broad sense, a detectable cancer has already seized the upper hand. This imbalance means it is essential to attack the cancer vigorously if it is to be brought back under the control of the immune system.

It is at this point that many health-conscious cancer patients who know the detrimental effects of conventional cancer treatment often make a critical mistake. Fearing side effects and a compromised immune system, they refuse all traditional chemotherapy and pursue alternative treatments only. Although many of these treatments boost the immune system, they have a marginal impact on the disease and seldom result in a cure or a lasting remission. The reason for this failure is that the cancer has already overwhelmed the immune system and become so strong that no simple immune stimulation can do any good by itself.

To start fighting cancer correctly, we must first weaken its grip by attacking the cancerous cells directly. This attack must, however, avoid damaging the immune system, which has already been compromised or suppressed enough to allow the cancer to grow. It is vital to remember that any long-lasting positive outcome to the disease of cancer presupposes a vigorous and sustained immunological response.

The key is finding cancer treatments that are effective at inflicting damage to cancer cells but do not significantly impair the immune system. Because both cancer cells and immune cells share the property of rapid proliferation, it is difficult to find a treatment that affects cancer but not the immune system. A magic bullet may not, however, be necessary; a treatment with differential effects on the two types of cells may be sufficient.

A combined, simultaneous treatment that targets cancer while enhancing the immune system, as we do in our integrative treatment model, is ideal. As cancer causes less and less immunosuppression in response to an effective treatment, the immune system has a chance to regain an upper hand, especially when it receives the nourishment of the right nutritional supplements, along with exercise and a positive attitude, key supports provided in our integrative clinic.

Once the immune system has regained complete control and immunoequilibrium with cancer is reestablished, a durable state of cancer remission can be achieved, sometimes lasting long enough that one must wonder if it is still there.

We know that conventional wisdom says that a stage 4 cancer is not curable. However, living *with* the existence of cancer with an immune system on guard is a situation that many of our patients have achieved. Many of these patients report that the integrative approach they follow leaves them feeling healthier than ever before.

When treating cancer, we must always consider the key convergence point of the integrative therapies. This brings us to chapter 3, where the antitumor response of the immune system works together with metronomic low-dose chemotherapy.

3

LESS IS MORE

The Benefits of Metronomic Low-Dose Chemotherapy

Every time my daughter begins a piano lesson, her teacher turns on a metronome, a mechanical device that produces an audible click at precise intervals that musicians use to set their tempo. As I listen to my daughter play, I am mindful of her efforts to maintain the proper rhythm, guided by the steady, reassuring swing of the metronome's pendulum.

It turns out that rhythm and pace also play a critical role in administering chemotherapy to cancer patients. Just as musicians can use a metronome to establish and maintain tempo, oncologists too can establish a "tempo" with consistent dosing frequency in chemotherapy that adjusts to the tumor's growing pace. Attention to rhythm and timing is no less important to effective cancer treatment than to a beautiful melody.

The Norton-Simon hypothesis, a now-proven principle of cancer chemotherapy developed by Dr. Larry Norton, a physician at Memorial Sloan-Kettering and the Evelyn H. Lauder Breast Center, and NCI statistician Richard Simon, explains that a tumor grows faster when it's small and slower when it's big.[1] A corollary to this is that tumor grows faster after chemotherapy, and if you don't time your treatment to this rhythm the tumor will grow back and eventually become resistant. By giving chemotherapy at lower doses more regularly, metronomic chemotherapy can catch these rebounding but more chemo-sensitive tumor cells and eradicate them with less toxicity. Dr. Norton once said, "I have a suspicion that we are using almost all the cancer drugs in the wrong way. For all I know, we may be able to cure cancer with existing agents." In my opinion, he is absolutely right.

WHAT IS METRONOMIC LOW-DOSE CHEMOTHERAPY (MLDC)?

Metronomic low-dose chemotherapy (MLDC) refers to the continuous, regularly spaced administration of low doses of chemotherapeutic drugs *without* extended rest periods between treatments.[2] The key to the success of MLDC protocols is their suitability for long-term, continuous administration.

This sustainability is also the main feature distinguishing MLDC from traditional maximum-tolerated dosage (MTD) chemotherapy, which typically can only be tolerated for a few cycles before serious side effects or the development of tumor resistance makes further treatment impossible.

The lower doses used in MLDC do more than minimizing side effects. Research on the mechanisms of MLDC suggests it works in two ways: by affecting cancer cells directly and, perhaps more importantly, by making the microenvironment less suitable for cancer growth.

One aspect of the microenvironment that is absolutely critical to the growth of a tumor is its ability to stimulate the production of new blood vessels, a process known as *angiogenesis*. MLDC has consistently been shown to suppress angiogenesis. Low doses of chemotherapy have also been found to work in concert with the immune system, enhancing its ability to fight cancer instead of shutting it down. Thus, the continual treatment of MLDC not only gives cancer cells less time to recover between treatment cycles; it enhances anticancer immune responses, suppresses cancer angiogenesis, and reduces the development of cancer drug resistance.

We can see parallels to MLDC in the boxing ring. For example, when a boxer is knocked down, the referee gives him until the count of ten to get back up and resume fighting. Imagine if the boxer who knocked his opponent down could resume fighting at the count of seven, while his opponent was still on his knees. In boxing as in fighting cancer, the chances of a successful outcome increase substantially when the opponent is not given a chance to recover. The denial of a meaningful recovery period is a central principle of metronomic low-dose chemotherapy.

Over the past two decades, standard chemotherapy treatment has hit a wall. Survival rates have reached a plateau, and fear of the severe side effects of the MTD approach has provoked widespread resistance to chemotherapy in cancer patients. MLDC represents a promising alternative approach to cancer chemotherapy, one that is both gentler and more effective than MTD. It merits more extensive consideration by oncologists as well as patients.

A BRIEF HISTORY OF MLDC

Around 2000, almost thirty years after the invention of chemotherapy, a group of scientists working at Dr. Judah Folkman's lab at Harvard University started to experiment on a different way of administering chemotherapy. Because Folkman's lab was the birthplace of anti-angiogenic cancer therapy, the approach of these scientists was to target the tumor vasculature that is essential for tumor survival and growth.

Folkman's colleagues consistently found that the administration of low doses of chemotherapy over prolonged, regular intervals resulted in the failure of vascular system to produce the new blood vessels needed by a growing tumor. These early studies also showed that the MLDC approach could reverse drug resistance that a tumor had developed earlier over the course of MTD chemotherapy. Follow-up work showed that MLDC worked much better in animals with intact immune systems than in immuno-deficient animals, suggesting that the mechanism behind the MLDC protocol involves the immune system.

Unfortunately, the attention of mainstream oncologists was riveted on the development of new cancer drugs at the time of Folkman's work and during the ensuing decade. The new drugs that were developed during this time went through the FDA approval process after testing with traditional MTD methods, which were much more well-known and therefore represented a safer route to regulatory approval.

In the profit-driven environment of the United States and much of the Western world, metronomic chemotherapy, despite the promise it showed in the Harvard trials, never really made it to the hospitals and clinics except for sporadic and relatively small studies. As we will see, metronomic chemotherapy is clearly the best way to administer cancer chemotherapy treatment. If it had been developed fully within the cancer treatment establishment, the landscape of cancer treatment might be very different today.

MTD METHODOLOGY AND THE DEVELOPMENT OF CONVENTIONAL CHEMOTHERAPY

To understand benefits of MLDC better, let's first discuss the conventional way of giving chemotherapy in maximum tolerated doses. The history of MTD chemotherapy probably dates back to 1964 when Skipper, Shabel, and Wilcox demonstrated the log-kill model of cancer cells in an exponentially growing leukemia cell line (L1210).[3] These scientists postulated that any given chemotherapy dose killed a constant fraction of cancer cells, regardless of the size of the tumor. With that in mind, they proposed that chemotherapy drugs should be given in doses as high as a patient could tolerate, because the highest tolerated dose would kill the greatest number of cancer cells. Moreover, they advised that this cycle should be repeated until the estimated number of cancer cells have fallen to zero. Clearly, the log-kill theory is quite compatible with the Western mentality that more is better.

Because of the assumption that more drugs kill more cancer cells, dosing was adjusted to the maximum level a patient could withstand. This log-kill theory and the MTD protocol it spawned came to dominate the cancer community's understanding of cancer growth and the best chemotherapy methods to treat it. Indeed, the MTD approach is still the dominant chemotherapy treatment method today.

According to the current drug development scheme, the MTD dose is determined in a "phase 1 clinical trial," in which patients in several cohorts are given increasingly higher doses of experimental drugs until unacceptable or life-threatening side effects—"dose-limiting side effects," or DLSs—are encountered. A drug dose below the DLS dose is empirically estimated and designated as the MTD because it does not trigger dose-limiting side effects in most people. Mild to severe side effects still occur, but they are considered acceptable so long as they are relatively infrequent and can usually be managed.

Built into the MTD scheme of chemotherapy is a long, essential interval of rest between each treatment cycle. These respites allow the patient to recover from side effects of MTD treatments such as bone marrow suppression, malnutrition associated with nausea, and so on. Unfortunately, a recovery period also benefits the cancer cells, especially those cells that are resistant to the drug or drug combination. Eventually, under the selection pressure of chemotherapy, most tumors become repopulated by drug resistant cancer cells, and the chemotherapy fails.

It must be admitted that part of the dominance of the MTD approach to cancer treatment is due to the fact it has had some success. MTD chemotherapy has been quite effective in the treatment of "liquid tumors," such as different forms of leukemia, as well as a limited number of chemo-sensitive solid tumors, such as testicular cancer and certain lymphomas. Cures of these malignancies with MTD treatments are common. Indeed, the survival probability for patients with the limited number of MTD-susceptible cancers actually increases when chemotherapy is administered at doses *above* MTD levels, which, unfortunately, is often associated with life-threatening side effects.

The administration of doses above MTD is called *myeloablative chemotherapy*, because it completely and permanently destroys ("ablates") a patient's bone marrow. This form of treatment, therefore, requires a bone marrow transplant as a rescue measure. However, even such high doses of chemotherapy sometimes fail to control aggressive malignancies. The possibility of recurrence has led to the daily or weekly drug administration after myeloablative therapy as maintenance therapy. This practice is very common in the treatment of pediatric cancer patients and employs the same general procedures as metronomic chemotherapy.

It is, however, important to emphasize that the success of MTD treatments has been limited. In particular, MTD therapy has met very limited success when used against most solid tumors at advanced stages. In part, this is because the log-kill theory does not apply well to solid tumors. In another part, it is likely related to overall immunosuppressive effects of the MTD treatments. Regardless of the cause, MTD chemotherapy has been labeled as only a palliative measure against stage 4 solid cancers by the oncology community. This label has attained the status of unalterable fact, and anyone who claims that advanced solid cancers *can* be cured or rendered in long-term remission by chemotherapy is instantly considered to be either naïve or a quack.

Once diagnosed, nearly all common cancers in their most advanced stages carry a median survival rate of one to three years, regardless of the treatment administered. The sense of defeat in the oncology community was reinforced when multiple studies showed high-dose myeloablative chemotherapy followed by bone marrow transplantation provided no survival advantage to patients with advanced breast and ovarian cancers.

Thankfully, myeloablative chemotherapy for solid tumors has now been permanently abandoned.

The pessimism spawned by the failure of MTD chemotherapy in advanced solid cancers became so pervasive that many patients with stage 4 cancers were sent to hospice immediately upon diagnosis, without receiving any treatment at all. This premature and unnecessary surrender occurred even though many studies showed that standard chemotherapy can at least improve the quality of life for terminal patients compared to no treatment at all.

A randomized study of four different combinations of MTD chemotherapy regimens for the treatment of stage 4 lung cancer was published several years ago in the *New England Journal of Medicine.* This study caused real despair among oncologists regarding the efficacy of MTD chemotherapy in treating lung cancer. The study showed that there was no difference in the four different high-dose regimens that were tested, and that only 20 percent of the patients showed any positive response to treatment when compared to patients who had no chemotherapy at all.

The insufficiencies of the log-kill model, upon which MTD chemotherapy is based, are clear from our current understanding of cancer biology. Most cancers, particularly solid tumors, do not grow exponentially; therefore, the log-kill model does not apply to them. Moreover, resistance to treatment builds up in treated patients as cancer cells mutate, gradually reducing their response to chemotherapy. Finally, tumor cells grow back between chemotherapy sessions, thereby reducing the chance of a steady, fractional reduction of tumor cell numbers as predicted by the model.

In all these cases, the prognosis did not improve until some biological agent targeting some aspect of the cancer microenvironment was introduced. Some monoclonal antibodies target tumor angiogenesis, while others also targeted cancer cells directly and activated the immune system. When these biological agents were included in a chemotherapy regimen, substantial improvements were observed.

Studies of the kind described above demonstrate the importance of the microenvironment to the growth and control of cancer. They suggest that more interventions can be done to alter the microenvironment of cancer cells, such as strengthening the immune system or decreasing the inflammation cancer causes, to improve cancer treatment responses.

ATTEMPTED BREAKTHROUGHS

During the 1970s, doctors Larry Norton, of Memory Sloan-Kettering Cancer Center, and George Simon, of the National Cancer Institute, developed an alternative model of cancer growth called the Norton-Simon hypothesis.[4] This theory was based on a population growth model originally proposed by Benjamin Gompertz, an eighteenth-century English statistician. The so-called Gompertizian model describes population growth that starts out exponential but then decreases to a plateau after a saturation of resources. The adaptation of the Gompertizian model to cancer growth states that cancer grows exponentially until it reaches a volume determined by the space and nutrients it can obtain from its microenvironment. Based on the Gompertizian model, Norton and Simon hypothesized that a tumor grows more rapidly when it's small, and more slowly when it's big. Therefore, chemotherapy should be given at high frequency to affect more cancer cells in their young, rapid growth phase. This is the basis of the concept of "dose dense chemotherapy," an approach that assumes the frequency, or dose density, of the chemotherapy administration is as important as the size of the dose itself in a single treatment.

However, like many scientific pioneers, Norton encountered so much doubt and hostility from the oncology community that he reportedly considered quitting oncology altogether. But he persevered and earned his sweet revenge in 2003, when the results of the landmark clinical trial CALGB 9741 were released.[5] This study compared two protocols with the same chemotherapy drug combinations and total drug dosages used but administered in different dosing frequency; one treatment group had drugs administered every two weeks, while the other received the same drugs every three weeks. The results of the study showed that the biweekly approach significantly improved the breast cancer patients' treatment outcomes, both in terms of reducing the risk of recurrence and breast-cancer-related mortality. Dr. Norton won the prestigious David A. Karnofski Award of American Society of Clinical Oncologists (ASCO) in 2004 in recognition of this work and the theory behind it.

Despite this breakthrough, fundamental changes to MTD-based cancer treatment have not yet occurred. Again, designing a better treatment schedule has fallen in priority to the glamorous business of inventing new cancer drugs, as once pointed out by Yale University professor and former NCI head Vincent DeVita. However, every cancer physician and researcher with a patient's true interest in mind should closely look at the principle and practice of MLDC and find out how making just small changes to our conventional way of giving chemotherapy can make a big difference in patient's treatment outcome and quality of life. We will now examine the MLDC alternatives to MTD treatments with special emphasis on the beneficial impacts of MLDC on cancer's microenvironment.

MLDC AND ANTIANGIOGENESIS

The groundbreaking work of metronomic chemotherapy started at the turn of the twenty-first century when it became increasingly clear that angiogenesis was a critical part of tumor growth and metastasis.

Angiogenesis is the formation of blood vessels that supply the oxygen and nutrients that cancerous (and all) tissues require for growth and survival. A classic experiment related to fighting cancer through disruption of the vascular processes necessary for tumor growth involved implanting a tumor into the cornea of a rabbit. Although corneal tissue typically does not have any blood vessels, new blood vessels arose in the cornea and grew into the implanted tumor. The oxygen and nutrients transported into the tumor by these new blood vessels allowed the tumor to grow. When, however, the advancing blood vessels were experimentally blocked, the tumor could not grow larger than about 0.4 mm. Much of current cancer research and treatment focuses on *antiangiogenesis*, or the development of angiogenesis inhibitors. Since the early 2000s there has been considerable hope that antiangiogenic drugs would be the "magic bullet" to inhibit the growth of cancer. Unfortunately, many antiangiogenics extend life for only a few months because of the development of drug resistance. In fact, there has been some speculation that the traditional administration of antiangiogenic agents in large doses may actually promote metastasis even though they inhibit the growth of the primary tumor.[6]

The exciting findings from experimental studies of metronomic chemotherapy are that the chemotherapy drugs, when administered in low doses regularly, have antiangiogenic activity without the trade-off of increased metastasis seen with MTD therapy. Moreover, metronomic administration of chemotherapy drugs may synergize with other direct antiangiogenic agents to induce complete tumor dormancy.[7]

Earlier work in the field of antiangiogenesis involved the administration of monoclonal antibodies that targeted either the growth factors stimulating vascular growth or the receptors for these growth factors. These studies showed treating cancer with these agents failed to induce tumor regression, although the growth rate of the tumor was reduced. A related study used an experimental model of neuroblastoma that was treated with vinblastine, a conventional chemotherapy drug. Low doses of vinblastine alone suppressed angiogenesis of an implanted neuroblastoma and temporarily slowed its growth. However, when the administration of low doses of vinblastine was combined with a monoclonal antibody to the receptor for the growth factor for angiogenesis, the "vascular endothelial growth factor" (VEGF) receptor, tumor reduction was dramatic and complete.

Dr. Browder demonstrated another promising metronomic regimen in animal models with low-dose cyclophosphamide given every six days. This treatment shrank tumors that had already become resistant to cyclophosphamide administered at MTD dosing.[8] When MLDC cyclophosphamide was combined with an anti-angiogenic agent, it induced complete and prolonged control of the chemo-refractory tumor. This study also showed that the mechanism of metronomic cyclophosphamide treatment was the induction of apoptosis in vascular endothelial cells, which was followed by apoptosis of tumor cells.

Further studies of the mechanisms of metronomic chemotherapy on angiogenesis suggested that the treatment either damages proliferating microvascular endothelial cells directly or suppresses circulating endothelial cells derived from bone marrow. Since tumors cannot grow without the nutrition and oxygen provided by blood vessels, one of the consequences of metronomic treatment is the induction of tumor dormancy.

Many chemotherapy drugs have been shown to have antiangiogenic impacts, especially when administered metronomically. Examples of antiangiogenic drugs include cyclophosphamide, vinblastine, paclitaxel, doxorubicin, and 5-FU. Generally speaking, these chemotherapy drugs are more effective in inducing apoptosis of vascular endothelial cells recruited by a tumor than in the tumor cells themselves. Therefore, only

lower doses of chemotherapy drugs are needed to achieve the antiangiogenic effect. This may be due at least partially to endothelial cells being
less resistant to chemotherapy drugs than cancer cells.

Vascular endothelial cells do, however, repopulate at a rapid pace,
using endothelial stem cells derived from bone marrow. Dr. McDonald
from UCSF vividly demonstrated this repopulation at the 28th Annual
German Cancer Congress in 2008. Using special microscopic imaging of
live tissues, he showed that endothelial cells lining the walls of the blood
vessel started sprouting and sending out growth processes from the basal
membrane after just one day of stopping an antiangiogenic drug. Within
just one week of stopping the antiangiogenesis treatment, the blood vessels and the blood supply to the tumor had been fully reestablished.[9]

The rapid repopulation of vascular tissue serving tumors shows that
frequent dosing of chemotherapy drugs is required to suppress tumor
angiogenesis. Although endothelial cells can still develop a resistance to
antiangiogenic therapy, they are much less prone to mutation than cancer
cells, and therefore require more time for the resistance to develop. The
antiangiogenic impact of the MLDC protocol is the basis of the synergy
between MLDC dosing and the use of various antiangiogenic agents.

An Israeli study showed that the same chemotherapy drug could have
opposite effects depending on whether it was administered following
MLDC or MTD protocols.[10] Dr. Shaked showed that doxorubicin *increased* angiogenesis in mice when given at maximum tolerated dosing
even though it suppressed tumor vascularization when administered metronomically. Blood serum from animals that had received MTD treatment
with doxorubicin was injected into half of a group of genetically identical
mice before both groups received tumor implants. Tumor growth and
metastasis was observed to be significantly higher in the group that had
received serum from MTD mice.

Taken together, these studies suggest that MTD chemotherapy increases tumor aggressiveness. This increase in aggressiveness, when
combined with the long interruptions in treatment characteristic of MTD
chemotherapy, is a major reason that MTD chemotherapy often fails so
quickly.

The stimulation of tumor proliferation and invasiveness by MTD
chemotherapy was also shown in a study by T. S. Chan that was reported
in the *Journal of Experimental Medicine* in 2016.[11] This study highlighted a specific mechanism that might explain in part why serum from

animals that had received MTD chemotherapy with doxorubicin increased the invasiveness of tumor cells implanted on other animals. Dr. Chan's study specifically investigated breast cancer stromal fibroblast cells, which are cells comprising the supporting framework or matrix of breast tumors. When exposed to such common chemotherapy drugs as Adriamycin, cyclophosphamide, or paclitaxel administered under an MTD protocol, these stromal cells secreted inflammatory cytokines that significantly enhanced the proliferation and invasiveness of nearby breast cancer cells. On the other hand, this tumor-promoting stromal reaction did not occur when the same drugs were administered under a MLDC protocol, even when the same quantity of drug was given under each regime.

MODULATION OF THE ANTICANCER IMMUNE RESPONSE

Another important mechanism of metronomic chemotherapy is its ability to regulate the antitumor immune response. It was recognized early on that metronomic chemotherapy was relatively ineffective against chemo-resistant cancer cells implanted into immunodeficient mice. If MLDC was ineffective in animals with a compromised immune system, it is clear that metronomic chemotherapy had to work through the immune system to achieve its antitumor effects.

Many studies have shown that metronomic chemotherapy enhances antitumor immune responses. One of the main mechanisms behind these impacts involves *T regulatory cells*, or *Treg cells*. Treg cells are part of the regulatory arm of the immune system. They reduce the intensity of immune responses and thereby play a vital role in preventing autoimmune diseases like lupus.[12] Metronomic low-dose chemotherapy reduces the number and activity of Treg cells, thereby freeing up other portions of the immune system to attack cancer cells.

Advanced cancers, on the other hand, have the opposite effect: they can "hijack" Treg cells, causing them to become overactive and to suppress nearly all aspects of an active antitumor response. This suppression clearly facilitates the proliferation and expansion of tumor cells. For example, it has been shown repeatedly that higher numbers of Treg cells in a cancer patient are associated with reduced numbers of cancer fighting immune cells in tumor tissues. These anticancer immune cells include NK cells and CD8 positive cytotoxic T lymphocytes.

One study used a mouse model of mesothelioma to show that depleting Treg cells prevented tumor cell repopulation during the rest period between cisplatin treatment cycles. Monoclonal antibodies against Treg cells were used to release the immune system from suppression by Treg cells. This study showed that Treg cells can contribute to tumor cell repopulation between treatment cycles and the development of chemoresistance by suppressing anticancer immune responses. [13]

Maximum tolerated dose chemotherapy has been shown to increase the activity of Treg cells, or the ratio of Treg to T effector cells. This finding sheds light on the true mechanism behind the failure of MTD chemotherapy. Specifically, it suggests that MTD chemotherapy fails not because *cancer cells* develop resistance to multiple chemotherapy drugs, but also because MTD chemotherapy *causes an increase in the number or activity of Treg cells.*

By contrast, MLDC reduces the number of Treg cells in tumor-bearing animals and human beings. The reduction is more prolonged and persistent in tumor tissues than in peripheral blood, probably due to the rapid repopulation of Treg cells from bone marrow. The reduction of Treg cells is also more pronounced than the reduction of the various effector T cells that are involved in the active immune response against the tumor. Thus, MLDC leads to a net gain in the immune response against cancer.

There is evidence that the mechanism behind the anticancer impact of MLDC administration of cyclophosphamide is associated with a reduction in the number of Treg cells and improved antitumor immune responses. Cyclophosphamide induces antitumor responses in both animal models and, in combination with vaccination, in human patients with metastatic melanoma or breast cancer. Cyclophosphamide also potentiated antitumor responses in hormone refractory prostate cancer patients. Peripheral blood samples from these patients showed a selective reduction in circulating Treg cells and improved antitumor immune responses.

Like cyclophosphamide, certain other chemotherapy drugs seem to exert an anticancer effect by reducing the number of Treg cells. For example, paclitaxel, an inhibitor of mitosis, given in metronomic doses with antigen-specific immunotherapy, reduced the number of Treg cells independently of its known role in suppressing angiogenesis. Paclitaxel also reduced the number of Treg cells in human patients with non-small cell lung carcinoma. [14]

Several studies have shown that various chemotherapeutic drugs increase the immune response to tumor vaccines. A mouse model of mammary carcinoma showed a small but significant immunomodulatory effect of a combination of doxorubicin or paclitaxel and antitumor vaccination. A human study of the combination of doxorubicin and tumor vaccine therapy showed low doses of both cyclophosphamide (200mg/m2) and doxorubicin (35mg/m2) enhanced the antibody responses to HER-2 vaccine. [15] Consistent with other dosing studies, this study also showed that higher doses of cyclophosphamide *suppressed* the vaccine response.

Any therapy that relies on a suppression of Treg cell production for its anticancer impact must come to grips with the fact that Treg cells repopulate themselves very rapidly—within forty-eight hours in some human studies. This makes metronomic dosing all the more important, as the population of Treg cells would otherwise quickly reestablish itself. Moreover, it has been speculated that even a transient suppression of Treg cells can trigger a lasting antitumor immune response. [16]

IMMUNE RESPONSES MEDIATED BY MYELOID DERIVED SUPPRESSOR CELLS

Another important target of metronomic chemotherapy is a type of immune suppressor cell called the *myeloid derived suppressor cell* (MDSC). Like Treg cells, the MDSC can suppress various aspects of both the innate and adaptive immune response to cancer.

Myeloid derived suppressor cells promote cancer by inhibiting the movement of other immune cells and by becoming more abundant as cancer progresses. A recent study found that MDSCs prevented activated T or B cells from entering tissues or lymph nodes in response to antigen stimulation. By removing an important molecule called L-selectin from these T or B cells, MDSC cells prevent them from entering cancerous tissue and mounting an immune response. [17] Moreover, MDSCs become more numerous as cancer progresses, likely playing an important role in the development of metastasis and the development of resistance to conventional treatment.

Unfortunately, there is a negative synergy between MTD chemotherapy and the natural increases in the MDSC population, because MTD therapy by itself increase the production of MDSCs. Thus, MTD can unleash a perfect storm in the immune system, releasing cancer from control of the acquired immune system. Metronomic chemotherapy, by contrast, has been consistently shown to suppress or decrease the number of MDSC cells in cancer patients.

Dendritic cells are another important type of immune cells that are enhanced by MLDC.[18] To reiterate, dendritic cells digest tumor fragments and present tumor antigens to T cells, thereby activating them to attack cancer cells. Researchers at Johns Hopkins University School of Medicine reported in January 2010 that oral cyclophosphamide administered according to an MLDC protocol enhanced antitumor immunity through effects that extend beyond suppression of Treg cells.[19] Specifically, they found that this treatment caused the emergence of tumor-infiltrating dendritic cells that were fully capable of priming antitumor T-cell responses but did not induce production of Treg cells.

Similar effects have been seen with other intravenous chemotherapy agents regarding enhancement of dendritic cell function in the antitumor response. Studies from the department of pathology at the University of Pittsburgh Medical Center found that nontoxic intravenously delivered chemotherapy drugs, including vinblastine, paclitaxel, azacytidine, methotrexate, and mitomycin C, can all stimulate CD80 expression of dendritic cells and enhance the ability of these cells to stimulate the proliferation of allogeneic T lymphocytes.[20] A related study from the same institution showed that low doses of paclitaxel and doxorubicin caused tumor cells to produce increased amounts of tumor-associated antigens. Human dendritic cells exposed to tumor cells pretreated with doxorubicin or paclitaxel developed an increased ability to activate tumor reactive T lymphocytes.

The production of tumor-specific antigens by tumors exposed to chemotherapy drugs illustrates a new approach to chemotherapy, one based on forcing cancer cells to produce antigens that mark them for destruction by the immune system. This approach is called "immunogenic tumor death." In this process, chemotherapy drugs induce cancer cells to express internal antigens that otherwise cannot be detected by the immune system. These chemo-induced cancer antigens include calreticulin (CRT) and heat shock protein (HSP), which are both examples of "damage-associated molecular patterns" (DAMPS). DAMPS molecules are efficient activators of the antigen-presenting cells that stimulate T cells to find cancer cells and induce their apoptosis. Although both high and low doses of chemotherapy can induce production of DAMPS and immunogenic cancer death, the more beneficial microenvironment conditioned by MLDC provides a much more suitable environment for an anticancer immune response than the MTD approach.

TARGETING TUMOR CELL REGROWTH

Under the Norton-Simon hypothesis, tumor cells grow faster after the initial round of chemotherapy because the decrease in tumor volume makes them more sensitive to chemotherapy drugs. The increased treatment frequency of the MLDC approach entails repeated attacks on the tumor at its most vulnerable stage. If the cancer cells can't recover after each treatment, they are much less likely to develop resistance to the chemotherapy. Compare this scenario to patients receiving MTD chemotherapy, who must take a break every two to four weeks to recover from the side effects of the treatment. This respite allows surviving cancer cells to absorb the hit and recover by proliferating at their fastest rate.

Remember the boxers? In that metaphor, the boxer still standing would be well advised to keep punching the one on the ground before he has a chance to recover and resume fighting.

According to doctors at the Instituto de Genética Experimental and the Facultad de Ciencias Médicas at the Universidad Nacional de Rosario in Rosario, Argentina, "The introduction of the 'maximum tolerated dose' in usual treatment protocols (and its concomitant overt toxicity) made necessary the imposition of rest periods between cycles of therapy—a practice that not only involves re-growth of tumor cells, but also growth of selected clones *resistant to the therapy.*"

As we know from the previous discussion, the inflammatory host response and rebound angiogenesis induced by MTD chemotherapy are the likely causes of this acceleration of tumor growth.

DOSE DENSITY AND DOSE INTENSITY

The dose density of a chemotherapy regime refers to the frequency with which chemotherapeutic drugs are administered. As has been seen, dose density has a powerful effect on therapeutic efficacy. Based on observed rates of tumor angiogenesis, chemotherapy should be administered at least once a week for a consistent antiangiogenic effect.[21]

The classic example of metronomic chemotherapy uses oral cyclophosphamide at 50mg, once a day. Although this treatment frequently results in the stabilization of a tumor that has become refractory to conventional treatment, it rarely results in remission when used by itself.[22] It is possible that oral cyclophosphamide has a good antiangiogenic effect when dose density is high, but this antiangiogenic impact is simply not strong enough to impact the tumor's viability.

Factors other than dose density affect the efficacy of metronomic chemotherapy. In particular, specific drug combinations and accumulative dose intensity—total chemotherapy dose per cycle—may also be important factors.

One example of an effective combination of chemotherapy agents is weekly administration of paclitaxel and carboplatin, a chemo regimen often used on advanced lung and gynecological cancers. A conventional regimen is to administer paclitaxel at 200mg/m2 and carboplatin at AUC 6 every twenty-one days. This regimen specified dose *intensity* but not dose *density*.

A regimen that combines dose density and accumulative dose intensity is weekly administration of paclitaxel at 70mg/m2 and carboplatin at AUC 2. This metronomic regimen can be more effective and more tolerable in cancer patients. The advantage of weekly metronomic chemotherapy over daily oral metronomic chemotherapy is that the weekly regimen entails a higher dose intensity while retaining enough frequency to prevent tumor angiogenesis. As a result, a weekly regimen is likely to be much more effective. The downside is that the weekly regimen will cause more side effects than the daily oral regimen, but it is still more tolerable than an MTD treatment.

Several groups researching dose density have examined a treatment regimen that combines MTD treatment followed by metronomic treatment, the so-called chemo-switch therapy.[23] The idea is that MTD is more potent in inducing cancer cell apoptosis, and metronomic treatment can suppress angiogenesis and reverse the activity of immune suppressor cells, such as Treg and MDSC cells, thereby preventing tumor regrowth. The initial results of chemo-switch therapy in animal studies have been very promising, with some reports of unprecedented high rates of tumor control. However, in my own clinical practice, when I was faced with a patient whose cancer had become refractory to multiple lines of chemotherapy, I just added a few days of oral cyclophosphamide or etoposide to the weekly chemotherapy regime. Usually, several weeks later, I found that the cancer in these patients had stabilized or even regressed.

In summary, high-dose chemo not only slugs the cancer with knockout punches, it also depresses the immune system and causes serious systemic and intra-tumor inflammation. Although the chemo initially knocks down the cancer, it grows back during the post-chemo recovery period, with the help of a weakened immune system reeling from the toxic effects of the chemotherapy and the inflammatory reaction that stimulates tumor angiogenesis and aggressiveness.

Unfortunately, the condition of a patient's immune system is essentially ignored during traditional MTD treatment. The only concession to normal physiology is the administration of a drug for nausea. Homeopathic medicine to boost the immune system, a topic addressed in chapter 4, is simply not available to most patients being treated in conventional cancer centers.

So patients receiving traditional protocols of MTD chemotherapy are put into double jeopardy by receiving too much chemotherapy, which weakens their immune system and renders them unable to receive more drugs successfully; it also makes them more susceptible to other illnesses.

By changing chemotherapy to metronomic dosing, all these problems can be largely avoided, and cancer treatment outcomes are significantly improved. Later in this chapter, we will present a clinical case to illustrate the effectiveness of this still novel approach to cancer treatment.

FORMS OF METRONOMIC CHEMOTHERAPY

Oral Metronomic Chemotherapy Agents

Oral chemotherapy agents, like cyclophosphamide and capecitabine, were the first agents studied with metronomic dosing. This was because pills are very easy to give to patients on a continuous basis, and the side effects of low-dose oral chemotherapy agents are usually minimal.

Over the years, various researchers have elucidated the basic mechanisms of metronomic chemotherapy, including antiangiogenesis and modulation of antitumor immune responses. Continuous dosing with such low-dose oral chemotherapy drugs has been studied most extensively in adults with multiple myeloma, and breast, ovarian, lung, and prostate cancer. We will discuss a few representative studies of oral metronomic chemotherapy here.

In 2002, researchers from the European Institute of Oncology in Milan, Italy, reported a study of low-dose oral methotrexate and cyclophosphamide in the treatment of patients with metastatic breast cancer who had already received extensive treatment.[24] Of sixty-three patients with refractory metastatic breast cancer, two developed complete remissions, ten developed partial remissions, and eight entered a period of stable disease after twenty-four weeks. Thus, 19 percent of these patients responded positively to some degree, and 31.7 percent either responded positively or stabilized. A drop in the levels of the growth factor stimulating angiogenesis (VEGF) was noted in the blood of patients with positive responses to treatment, and this decrease was identified as the mechanism underlying the response. A different mechanism was identified in a 2007 French study of end-stage cancer patients who were also treated with a metronomic regimen of cyclophosphamide. The function of anticancer T lymphocytes and NK cells was restored in treated patients, and this response was attributed to a decrease in the number of Treg cells and other cells known to suppress the immune response.[25]

An Italian review of the results of 153 patients with advanced breast cancer who were treated between 1997 and 2003 once again showed that metronomic oral chemotherapy can induce prolonged clinical benefits in patients with metastatic breast cancer.[26] Over 15 percent of the patients in the study achieved control of their cancer for at least twelve months, and the median time to progression for these patients was twenty-one months. One patient maintained complete remission forty-two months after the therapy had been discontinued.

Two studies explored the synergy of metronomic oral chemotherapy and antiangiogenesis therapy. A 2008 study reported in the journal *Breast Cancer* examined the response of patients with advanced breast cancer to a treatment combining oral metronomic cyclophosphamide and capecitabine with bevacizumab, a monoclonal antibody to vascular endothelial growth factor (VEGF) that suppresses vascularization of tumors. In response to this treatment, 2 percent of patients achieved complete remission, 46 percent achieved partial remission, and 41 percent achieved a stable disease state.[27] A similar study conducted in 2007 at the University of Minnesota combined bevacizumab and low-dose metronomic oral cyclophosphamide in ovarian cancer patients with a history of five or more cycles of failed chemotherapy. Of the fifteen patients who could be evaluated, two had a complete remission and six had a partial remission. The author concluded that this treatment provides significant promise for heavily pretreated ovarian cancer patients, with an overall response rate of 53 percent and no significant toxicity.[28] Capecitabine is another oral chemotherapy drug that is suitable for metronomic chemotherapy. In a study published in *Lancet* in April 2013, Dutch researchers reported that colorectal cancer patients who had been treated with MTD chemotherapy achieved prolonged progression-free survival with minimal side effects and no deterioration of quality of life when put on maintenance treatment with capecitabine and bevacizumab.[29]

A similar study published in *Journal of Clinical Oncology* in 2008 reported that breast tumors either shrank or stabilized in almost 90 percent of the treated patients. Higher baseline circulating endothelial cells correlated with overall response, clinical benefit, and improved progression-free survival. In this case, the treatment consisted of a combination of oral metronomic cyclophosphamide and capecitabine plus intravenous bevacizumab.[30]

Another therapeutic approach involves hypoxia inducible factor 1 (HIF-1). Hypoxia inducible factor 1 has been found in many human cancers, and in their metastases. It is associated with the induction of genes implicated in angiogenesis, tumor metabolism, invasion, and metastasis, and its presence is associated with poor patient survival. Therefore, the inhibition of HIF-1 has attracted study as a potential strategy for cancer therapy.

In a study published in *Clinical Cancer Research* in 2011, researchers found that daily, low-dose oral topotecan reduced HIF-1 expression with an associated decrease in the levels of two factors (VEGF and GLUT-1 mRNA) associated with tumor blood flow and the permeability of tumor blood vessels. This effect was achieved in seven of ten patients after one cycle. This study indicated that oral metronomic topotecan may contribute to the tumor control through suppression of HIF-1 expression and associated tumor angiogenesis. [31]

Single Agent Intravenous Metronomic Chemotherapy

Of all intravenous chemotherapy agents, paclitaxel is one of the best studied. In a randomized phase 3 trial, a weekly paclitaxel dose density was compared to a dose density of once every three weeks on a group of patents with HER-2 positive breast cancer. It was found that weekly administration of paclitaxel was superior to once every three weeks; weekly versus once every three weeks administration resulted in response rates of 42 percent and 29 percent, respectively, and respective times to disease progression of nine versus five months. Perhaps most importantly, patient survival with weekly treatments was twice that for treatment every three weeks, increasing from twelve to twenty-four months.

In a meta-analysis of over 1,700 patients and seven studies, patients corroborated the results of the previous study. Weekly paclitaxel treatments were associated with significant survival advantages as well as reductions in serious adverse events from neutropenia, neutropenic fever, and peripheral neuropathy. The advantage of administering paclitaxel on a weekly versus once every three-week basis was also seen in an early breast cancer adjuvant and neoadjuvant chemotherapy trial. Weekly metronomic paclitaxel treatments were found to have stronger antiangiogenesis effect than once-every-three-weeks MTD chemotherapy, as well as a stronger immune regulatory effect.

In an article published in *Molecular Therapy*, researchers from Taiwan University Hospital found that a metronomic paclitaxel regimen was synergistic with antigen specific DNA vaccine in delaying tumor growth and preventing metastasis.

Combination Metronomic Chemotherapy

Combination metronomic chemotherapy is often needed because single agents have a narrow spectrum of effective dose intensity. Because of this restriction, single agent oral or intravenous chemotherapy often results in more tumor stabilization than tumor reduction in clinical trials. Such outcomes are associated with a shortened duration of response. Therefore, large or aggressive tumors usually require combination metronomic chemotherapy, such as weekly Taxol and carboplatin, with or without bevacizumab.

Combination chemotherapy explores synergies of individual chemo-therapy drugs in targeting both the tumor microenvironment and tumor cells directly. Such a dual focus can lead to a more rapid and durable tumor response. However, due to the accumulation of side effects from individual drugs, toxicity from combination chemotherapy can be significant and more difficult for weak patients to tolerate. Therefore, as described in chapter 4, supportive care is crucial for patients undergoing multi-agent chemotherapy.

Along with my former colleague, Dr. Chue, I first reported a metro-nomic multiagent chemotherapy protocol for patients with refractory metastatic pancreatic cancer at an ASCO meeting in 2006. This treatment consisted of weekly paclitaxel, oxaliplatin, leucovorin, and 5-FU (POLF). Four patients with advanced pancreatic cancer were treated with the POLF regimen, three of whom had previously failed one or two lines of chemotherapy. After just two weeks of metronomic POLF treatment, all four patients experienced a dramatic improvement, with a mean reduction of the pancreatic cancer marker CA-19.9 of 80 percent. All four patients were considered to be in partial remission after a three-month course of treatment. One of these patients, who initially came to us on a stretcher with widely metastatic disease, eventually recovered, went back to work, and survived for more than six years.

This protocol has since benefited many more patients in our practice.

In the 2008 World Congress of Lung Cancer held in Hawaii, I reported on fourteen consecutive patients with advanced non-small cell lung cancer (stage 3b or 4), These patients were treated from 2002 through 2007 with a first line metronomic chemotherapy consisting of weekly Taxol and carboplatin, with or without bevacizumab. All of the patients received complementary supportive care from naturopathic providers.

By the standards of conventional MTD treatments, these patients were expected to have only a 20 percent to 30 percent chance of response to treatment, and a nine- to twelve-month survival rate. Remarkably, all of our patients responded to the metronomic protocol, and 50 percent of the responders eventually achieved complete remission after treatment durations ranging from six months to a year. Tumors were observed to shrink continuously during treatment. At the five-year follow-up, median survival was thirty-six months, and the five-year median survival rate was 25 percent. Both numbers tripled the current statistics for lung cancer survival following conventional MTD chemotherapy. Equally remarkable was the fact that the treatment was very well tolerated, causing only a minimal incidence of mild side effects.

A COMMONSENSE AND SCIENTIFIC APPROACH TO CANCER TREATMENT

As we have seen, it is not just common sense to give chemotherapy at lower doses and more frequently. The science bears this out, too. Metronomic chemotherapy is a multi-targeted cancer treatment that kills tumor cells directly while triggering the body's antitumor immune reaction at the same time.

In summarizing the promise of metronomic low-dose chemotherapy, it is appropriate to cite a March 2015 article in *Cancer Letters*. This article was titled "Metronomic Chemotherapy: An Attractive Alternative to Maximum Tolerated Dose Therapy that Can Activate Antitumor Immunity and Minimize Therapeutic Resistance," and was coauthored by Irina Kareva, David J. Waxman, and Giannoula Lakka Klement, all affiliated with the Tufts Medical Center in Boston. The article highlighted the following five empirically observed effects of MLDC:

1. Metronomic chemotherapy involves administering lower doses of chemotherapeutic drugs at more frequent intervals.
2. Lower dosage allows targeting supporting tumor stroma without selecting for resistant cells, unlike cases of antibiotic resistance.
3. Lower dosage and more frequent administration allow preservation and maintenance of antitumor immunity.
4. Metronomic chemotherapy yields long-term improved clinical outcome despite slower initial decreases in tumor size.
5. Cancer is a disease of both tumor cells and their microenvironment.

I have seen the positive results of this "less is more" protocol in my practice for many years, and I believe these five points fairly summarize the promise of MLDC at the present time.

CHEMOTHERAPY—DON'T ABANDON IT; IMPROVE IT!

The knowledge acquired in studies of metronomic chemotherapy, combined with the clinical experience we continue to accumulate, will lead to a change in the design of anticancer therapies. The core function of immune modulation by MLDC can be synergistic with all the new therapies that target the microenvironment of the tumor. These new therapies include antiangiogenic therapy, immunotherapy, targeted therapy, and integrative therapies that are anti-inflammatory and immune-supportive.

The central theme of all these treatment modalities is to support the body's own fighting power against cancer: the immune system. Unfortunately, the condition of a patient's immune system is essentially ignored during a traditional course of treatment. Even now, with an increasing understanding of the importance of the immune system in cancer control, the general oncology community still does not recognize the immunosuppressive effect of conventional high-dose chemotherapy.

Patients and physicians alike often mistakenly think that supporting a patient's white blood cell or neutrophil production with hematopoietic growth factors is a form of support for the immune system. Unfortunately, this belief is mistaken, at least in terms of the effect on cancer. Unlike NK cells and T cells, white blood cells play a minor role controlling cancer, even though their ability to control bacterial infections is crucial.

Diet, supplements, exercise, and mind-body medicine can all boost the body's anticancer immune responses. Unfortunately, these factors are considered less a mainstay of cancer treatment than a sparingly used garnish to conventional treatment in most cancer centers. We will discuss these integrative factors further in chapter 4.

Although the clinical development of MLDC over the last decades has been stagnant for various reasons, the rapidly developing field of cancer immunotherapy, particularly immune checkpoint inhibitor therapies, has sparked a new interest in MLDC as an adjunct to these new therapies.

In comparison to MTD chemotherapy, MLDC is more adaptive, integrative, and holistic. It affords the option of a more gentle and effective approach to cancer therapy. It suggests the possibility of transforming cancer into a chronic disease, one we may be able to control to allow people to live longer, fuller, and qualitatively healthier lives.

As we continue to search for scientific answers to the challenges of cancer, we have much to learn from the wisdom of spiritual teachings, especially those that proclaim that evil is overcome not by might nor by power, but by the spirit within us.

Putting our trust in big guns and a knockout approach has brought us neither short-term comfort nor lasting good health. While we all want peace in our lives, we often forget that it starts on a cellular level. Life begins as a single cell, so why should healing be any different? When our body is at peace, reacting harmoniously to an integrative treatment, our chances of healing increase exponentially. Success depends on the preservation and strengthening of our own innate healing power.

CASE STUDY

Ted is a seventy-three-year-old retired helicopter pilot who has now survived recurrent metastatic lung cancer for eight years. He was first diagnosed with what was then thought to be an early-stage, left-sided, non-small cell lung cancer, after experiencing a relentless cough and chest pain. He underwent a surgical resection of his left upper lung (lobectomy) and was told that the cancer had been completely removed.

Nine months later, however, a CT scan showed enlarged lymph nodes in the mediastinum (the area in the chest between the lungs that contains the heart, the trachea, the esophagus, and the great vessels entering and leaving the heart). A PET scan confirmed that these were lymph nodes involved with a highly aggressive metastatic cancer, consistent with recurrent lung cancer. Even worse, there was evidence that the cancer had spread to Ted's right shoulder.

Ted's oncologist told him he was not a candidate for another surgery or radiation. He did, however, offer a chemotherapy treatment plan that would be given every three weeks for a maximum of six to eight times. He was told his life expectancy with this treatment was between nine and twelve months. Without it, he was told his life expectancy was two to six months.

After hearing about the side effects, he would probably have to endure, Ted opted for the second choice: go home and get his affairs in order. His daughter, who then worked as a reporter at a local newspaper, had read a story about a stage 4 lung cancer patient I had treated. This patient had also been given no hope but had survived for over five years at that time. Ted's daughter and wife then convinced him to see me for a second opinion.

I was quite confident I could help Ted. I had in fact just reported to the International Lung Cancer Congress on a series of stage 4 lung cancer patients I had treated in my clinic from 2003 to 2008. My confidence was based on the fact I had been able to control disease in 100 percent of these patients and had tripled their survival time compared to conventional treatment.

I immediately started Ted on a metronomic weekly chemotherapy regime of Taxol and carboplatin, and added weekly cetuximab, a monoclonal antibody targeting the epidermal growth factor receptor on the surface of cancer cells. Previous clinical trials using cetuximab with MTD chemotherapy had been disappointing, with minimal improvement over chemotherapy alone. However, cetuximab has a unique function called antibody dependent cytotoxicity (ADCC), which works like a bridge between the tumor and cancer-fighting immune system cells, such as macrophages and natural killer cells. These cells, once bound to cetuximab through a receptor on their surface, called a Fc receptor, can mount an attack on cancer cells at close range.

While it was not surprising to me that the immunosuppressive impact of MTD therapy had eliminated a positive immune response to cetuximab, it made perfect sense to me to add cetuximab to a metronomic chemotherapy regimen. Cetuximab seemed a promising addition to MLDC therapy because of its stimulation of the antitumor immune response.

Before treating Ted, I had already successfully treated several other cancer patients with this regimen. Ted and his family agreed to the treatments right away, even though it meant that he and his wife would have to drive four hours round trip every week. Other than mild fatigue and a skin rash, typical of cetuximab treatment, the treatment went smoothly. Ted tolerated the treatment very well. Twelve weeks later, a repeat PET-CT scan showed that the metastatic cancer in the middle of his chest and right shoulder was almost gone. He continued the treatment for another twelve weeks, and a second scan showed the cancer activities in these areas had completely disappeared.

Since Ted was still tolerating the treatment well and could breathe more easily with all cancer activity gone, we decided to give him another round of low-dose chemo to consolidate the treatment results. After a third PET-CT scan showed that he remained in complete remission, he took a whole month off, and started a monthly maintenance of chemo, which I recommended to prevent cancer recurrence.

Ted followed this maintenance schedule religiously for about a year, and after several scans showed that his cancer remained in remission, he requested to extend the interval of the maintenance treatment from four to eight months. Six months later, a PET-CT scan showed that his cancer had returned to the same areas, although less aggressively than before. Ted immediately restarted the same metronomic low-dose chemotherapy regimen and, twelve weeks later, a scan showed his cancer had disappeared again. Ted's cancer returned about four years after the initial diagnosis; he was treated again with the same metronomic regime, and a third complete remission was obtained. Ted is now, four years after this third treatment, still in remission while maintaining a monthly maintenance treatment. During these four years, Ted had to deal with a flare up of his COPD, as well as back surgery to eliminate his sciatic nerve pain. But he rarely missed any treatments despite chemo, COPD, and sciatica surgery. He also finally finished his long-term project of building his own home, a project he had started before he was diagnosed.

This case illustrates that MLDC can be tolerated over a prolonged period of time to gradually induce remission of cancers that are difficult to treat. It can work well with immunotherapy to activate the body's native cancer fighting power to achieve a durable, long-lasting remission. It is suitable for long-term maintenance chemotherapy treatment. When cancer does relapse, it can be used repeatedly to re-induce remission, as it is much harder for cancer to develop resistance to this form of treatment, as we discussed earlier in this chapter.

THE WAVE OF THE FUTURE

So is metronomic low-dose chemotherapy counterintuitive or just plain smart? Over the past two decades, MTD chemotherapy treatment has hit a wall as people have recognized its severe side effects, including immuno-suppression, which leads to infection as well as uninhibited cancer growth.

We know that metronomic low-dose chemotherapy is a multi-targeted therapy that exerts both direct and indirect effects on tumor cells and their microenvironment. It can inhibit tumor angiogenesis, stimulate anticancer immune response, and induce tumor dormancy. By using lower doses of various chemotherapeutic drugs *without* extended rest periods to target activated endothelial cells in tumors, the side effects of traditional chemo-therapy are minimized. This consistent treatment also allows for more accurate dose adjustments based on close monitoring of a patient's condi-tion. Practitioners using MLDC believe that it works *with* the immune system, enhancing its ability to fight cancer, rather than shutting down the immune response.

That being said, MLDC is not a miracle cure. It is simply a relatively new approach that holds great promise. But cancer patients who have undergone conventional treatment will testify to the horribly debilitating side effects of MTD, side effects which often cause suspension of treat-ment. Conversely, those who have experienced MLDC will testify to its relative gentleness.

With metronomic low-dose chemotherapy, it is possible to obtain ther-apeutic effects that go a long way to transforming cancer into something we can live with. Our pragmatic, therapeutic objective now might be better focused on shrinking tumors gradually while building up our im-munity through a well-balanced approach to treatment.

All modalities of care that support our immune system merit consider-ation in a customized MLDC program. The choice of modalities is the prerogative of individual doctors, informed patients, and their caregivers. Although cancer chemotherapy is still dominated by MTD methods, equivalent "metronomically oriented" treatment protocols do exist. Re-searchers need to conduct more studies on MLDC to bring it into main-stream oncology.

In light of the weight of the scientific evidence supporting the low-dose approach, as well as the fixation of conventional oncologists on the MTD approach to treatment, the stakes for a cancer patient are high. As a patient, you must ask questions, do your homework, and seek advice from healthcare practitioners and others you trust—until you can finally make decisions for yourself. Challenge your oncologist to consider ideas, which may be new to him or her and their practice. From seeing the benefits of MLDC on a daily basis, I believe the switch to MLDC needs to happen sooner rather than later.

4

EAST MEETS WEST

The Value of Integrative Cancer Therapies

Like many patients I have treated over the years, Bickley Barich received high-dose chemotherapy at a local hospital for her stage 4 metastatic ovarian cancer. But after three years of heavy treatment, Bickley's health was not improving, and the cancer spread to her chest and lungs causing bouts of painful coughing. Her oncologist told her there was nothing more he could do, that she should take care of her affairs and find a good hospice. Soon thereafter, she found my clinic, and we began a program of weekly metronomic low-dose chemotherapy, along with antiangiogenic therapy with bevacizumab and immune supportive therapy, accompanied by high doses of intravenous vitamin C and other supplements. This new integrative treatment plan elicited the best response she had ever had, eventually taking her all the way to complete remission.

That was more than ten years ago, during which time Bickley continued taking maintenance antiangiogenic therapy, intermittent chemotherapy, and supplements that kept her immune system strong. She also kept up her improved diet, an exercise plan, and, equally important—a hopeful attitude about life. She learned that a cancer diagnosis does not have to stop her life, that with appropriate treatment and a strong immune system, cancer can be turned into a chronic illness one can live with. Bickley came to personify the multifaceted benefits of diet, nutrition, and supplements, as well as certain elements of traditional Chinese medicine.

Although Bickley sadly passed away recently after fifteen years with our clinic, her story exemplifies what can happen when East meets West, when a therapy integrates metronomic low-dose chemotherapy and naturopathic medicine to boost the immune system and control cancer. This regimen of integrative therapy not only allowed Bickley to extend her life, but to make it a life worth living. During her cancer treatment, she happily witnessed the marriage of both of her daughters and the births of two grandchildren.

Bickley's case demonstrates the importance of enhancing the immune system with integrative cancer therapies. You have already seen that metronomic low-dose chemotherapy attacks cancer directly while also preserving and stimulating the immune system. We have used this combined approach successfully on a wide range of cancers, and our patient survival rates significantly surpass national averages.

WHAT IS INTEGRATIVE CANCER THERAPY?

Integrative cancer therapy generally refers to a variety of physical, emotional, and spiritual measures that complement conventional chemotherapy, which targets cancer growth directly. Integrative cancer therapies optimize a patient's nutritional status and immune function at the same time as they decrease cancer-induced inflammation and angiogenesis. Specific measures that can be a part of integrative therapy include: a careful selection of scientifically proven vitamins, minerals, and supplements; advanced nutritional guidance; an individually tailored exercise program; mindfulness-based stress reduction; yoga and meditation; art, music, and writing therapies; and other measures that make the cancer's microenvironment less suitable for the growth and metastasis of cancer cells.

When any or all of these integrative therapies are introduced in conjunction with metronomic low-dose chemotherapy, they form a synergistic model of cancer care, a model that we have employed in our clinic with consistent success.

The details of integrative cancer therapy vary from patient to patient, depending on numerous factors, but the objectives always include improved nutritional status, enhanced immune function, and the strengthening of tolerance of conventional treatments. The last objective, boosting tolerance, bears additional comment, because some people think increased tolerance is the main objective of integrative therapy. Although integrative cancer therapy does reduce the severity of treatment side effects and controls cancer-related symptoms, it also improves the outcome of conventional treatments while enhancing a cancer patient's overall quality of life.

WHY DO WE NEED IT?

Cancer is a much bigger problem than can be addressed by treatments that merely target tumors. As we have seen with the maximum tolerated dosing (MTD) approach, intensive chemotherapy can quickly overwhelm a patient. Even the MLDC, which always entails lower doses of chemotherapy drugs, can take a toll on a patient. Cancer impacts the whole person, body, mind, and spirit, and all of these elements must be addressed for the healing to be deep and lasting.

Many conventional oncologists have very little knowledge of cancer therapies outside of what they have read in university textbooks and traditional Western oncology journals. When asked about the role of diet, nutrition, and complementary medicine, such doctors often dismiss these measures en masse as useless, a waste of time, or, at best, nothing important. Many patients have encountered this patronizing kind of response from close-minded oncologists. When one of my patients with stage 4 lung cancer asked her previous oncologist about what dietary supplements she should consider, she was told, "You can take a Flintstone vitamin if you like, but it won't make any difference." Responses of this type show just how oblivious some oncologists can be about their patients' need for comprehensive advice and support, including emotional support, in their fight for survival.

Intuitively, and often despite their doctor's disinterest, many patients start to pay closer attention to their lifestyles after being diagnosed with cancer. This analysis usually includes an honest examination of their diet and nutrition, their approach to reducing stress, the quantity and quality of their sleep, and their exercise habits. A cancer diagnosis is a major wake-up call. In the wake of a cancer diagnosis, sometimes for the first time in their life, patients become intensely interested in learning about anything they can do to improve their health, their chance of survival, and their quality of life.

Anxious patients begin to look for help wherever they can find it, online, and from family and friends. It is very important that they get the right guidance at this time, because the topics of cancer and cancer therapy include an astounding amount of dangerous misinformation.

In my experience, patients who start with a good integrative treatment plan at the very beginning fare much better than those who start later, especially if the patient has already started undergoing MTD chemotherapy. This is because the immune system, which holds the key to cancer control, needs to be preserved and stimulated early on while MTD chemotherapy can suppress the immune system and promotes drug resistance. Integrative therapies are also tolerated much better than MTD treatments, which translates into a high degree of patient compliance with the treatment plan.

CANCER'S IMPACT ON THE WHOLE PERSON

Even though cancer arises in a single organ, its impact is like an earthquake: although damage is worst at the epicenter, shock waves ripple through the entire body, causing damage in distant areas. Human organ systems are so intricately interconnected that a strong impact to any single system inevitably disrupts all other systems to some degree. Let us now look at some of the interrelated impacts of cancer on the whole person.

Physical Aspects

Let's begin with some of the direct physical effects of cancer. The most direct physical damage is a result of the aggressive, uncontrolled growth of cancer cells, which compromises or blocks the function of the affected organ and nearby organs. Tumor growth can also cause pain in surrounding nerves, swelling due to inflammation, or bleeding if blood vessels are invaded.

In addition to the mechanical impact of tumor growth, cancer disrupts biochemical pathways and communication among various organ systems. The mediator of this disruption is the *inflammatory response* that cancer invariably invokes. Ironically, destructive cancer-induced inflammatory responses are actually the body's misguided attempts to get rid of the disease, but end in promoting the cancer growth and the development of treatment resistance due to multiple factors such as stimulation of angiogenesis and suppression of the immune system.

Naturally produced chemicals called *cytokines* mediate the inflammatory response, as well as other symptoms commonly seen in cancer patients, such as weight loss, fatigue, and depression. In turn, these responses trigger a cascade of mind/body interactions that can create a vicious cycle of inflammation and psychological debilitation.[1]

For example, the inflammatory cytokines tumor necrosis factor alpha (TNFα), Interleukin-6, and Interleukin-1 are all involved in a cancer-induced wasting syndrome called *cachexia*. Cachexia is characterized by steady, unrelenting weight loss and muscle wasting. These same three inflammatory cytokines are also implicated in depression and fatigue.[2]

Weight loss is very common in cancer patients. Indeed, unexplained weight loss is one of the first signs of cancer, often triggering the examination that leads to an initial diagnosis. When significant weight loss occurs, it contributes to a decreased sense of well-being and adds greatly to a patient's distress over his or her cancer diagnosis. The weight loss of cachexia is often incorrectly seen as a result of uncontrolled cancer growth. Even in some scientific circles, there are those who believe that cancer "steals" nutrients from the body, leading to nutritional deficiency and weight loss. However, it is now known that cancer causes a systemic inflammation, which leads to a catabolic state that causes weight loss regardless of the amount of food ingested or the nutritional consumption of the tumor.[3] (A *catabolic physiological state* is a hormone-induced disruption of metabolism that maximizes energy production by transforming muscle tissue and other proteins into glucose, and inhibits metabolic processes leading to tissue maintenance or growth.)

The major loss of weight caused by this cancer-induced catabolic state is often associated with a loss of lean body muscle mass that compounds other problems, such as fatigue, depression, anxiety, as well as a compromised immune system. This physical and mental dysfunction is known as *cachexia syndrome*, and it is common in patients with end-stage disease. Cachexic weight loss also decreases quality of life, decreases a patient's ability to function in a normal manner, increases the incidence of complications, and leads to disruptions in the treatment schedule.

Weight loss is an important warning sign of nutritional deficiency that, if untreated, can be deadly. It is estimated that 20 percent of terminal cancer patients actually die from malnutrition and not from the cancer itself. Moreover, almost 50 percent of patients who die from cancer were malnourished before they died. Malnutrition plays a major role in the death of up to 85 percent of the patients who die from head and neck cancer and esophageal cancer.

Malnutrition compromises various disease-fighting mechanisms of the body, from immune system function to the healing ability of tissue, as well as the regeneration of blood-producing cells in the bone marrow. All of these factors are important in the process of cancer treatment and recovery.

Mental/Emotional Aspects

Being diagnosed with cancer and going through treatment is often associated with the development of depression or an exacerbation of preexisting depression. Major depression is estimated to occur in at least 15 percent to 25 percent of all cancer patients. This depression is often associated with other psychological symptoms such as anxiety, stress, and fear.

Various factors other than psychological issues may contribute to the development of depression. When given in high doses for cancer treatment, interferon alpha is known to cause depression. Chronic inflammation induced by cancer can also suppress the immune response, sometimes leading to the reactivation of an occult herpes viral infection that worsens chronic fatigue and depression. Some chemotherapy drugs can directly increase the production of inflammatory cytokines, like IL-6, which when elevated persistently can lead to muscle wasting and difficulties with walking. Impaired locomotor ability only exacerbates problems associated with fatigue and weight loss, increasing the likelihood of the development of depression.

Depression can also magnify and worsen some common physical problems associated with cancer, such as pain, fatigue, loss of appetite, insomnia, and excessive sleepiness. Severe depression can cause behavioral problems, including loss of interest in life, frequent crying, and isolation from friends and family.[4] Cognitive symptoms, including difficulty concentrating, struggling to make decisions, memory problems, and deeply negative or even suicidal thoughts can also arise.

In a clinical setting, it is not uncommon for depression to be a major roadblock in a patient's path to recovery. Depression can cause indecisiveness in choosing a treatment option or premature withdrawal from an ongoing and effective treatment. Depression does not only affect the patient. It snares the families that are trying to help that person. A severely depressed patient is significantly more challenging for personal and professional caregivers. Good intentions often turn into frustration on the part of the caregiver, which in turn causes more depression in the patient.

Depression is known to be a strong predictor of treatment responses and outcomes for cancer patients. A 2010 German meta-analysis of studies that examined the relationship between depression and cancer outcomes found that a diagnosis of depression and higher levels of depressive symptoms, both before and after cancer diagnosis, were associated with a significantly shorter post-diagnosis survival time.[5]

Spiritual and Social Aspects

Although cancer's primary effects on a patient are clearly physical, we know from years of research and clinical experience that a cancer diagnosis doesn't take long to affect the spirit and social status of a patient. These spiritual effects have direct consequences for the short- and long-term prognosis of patients and their respective families and communities.

While almost all cancer patients complain of fatigue and varieties of other psychological symptoms, they are often only offered simple but ineffective advice. What cancer patients have not been advised by the well-meaning suggestions of "Take more naps if you're tired," or "Drink a protein shake if you can't eat"? At best, such advices address symptoms without delving deeper into the causes and a more detailed plan to address them. Many oncologists do recognize the significance of these problems but feel powerless in their ability to address them with limited knowledge and tools in their toolbox. When the frustration for these unsolvable problems builds up, physicians as well as the patients are all more likely to give up the treatments, often prematurely. This is often the time patients like Bickley Barich are told that there is nothing more can be done and that it is time to take care of affairs and find a good hospice.

Fortunately, Bickley had the spiritual energy to pursue a better option as well as the social support to make the most of it. These factors carried her for many productive years beyond what she had thought was possible. I hope you will have the same drive and resources if you are diagnosed with cancer. I hope you will be able to find a physician who provides a rich menu of integrative therapies to treat the cancer, as well as to promote good overall health and quality of life. These are the fundamental goals of integrative oncology.

Now let us continue our exploration of integrative cancer therapy starting with the ancient Chinese wisdom about the yin and yang of diseases and the medicines used to treat them.

THE ART OF *FU ZHENG QU XIE*

According to traditional Chinese medicine, the essence of a basic strategy for treating cancer or any disease is *fu zheng qu xie*, which translates roughly to "strengthening the body's positive force to fend off the negatives that promote disease." *Zheng* is often represented by "*Qi*," which denotes life energy and host resistance, factors more commonly referred to as "immunity" in the West. Thus, genuine *Qi* is the foundation of the human body's immune function, which is the key to any strategy for controlling cancer. It implies that the success of any external intervention to eliminate the disease must first support the body's own disease-fighting capabilities.[6]

Ancient Chinese wisdom confirms what we know today, that fortifying the body's immune system and boosting its nutritional, physical, and spiritual status are essential factors in fighting cancer. We know that a strong immune system response to cancer holds the key to long-lasting cancer remission. Research has shown that treating cancer with metronomic low-dose chemotherapy is associated with stronger cancer immune response and in our experience longer-lasting remissions in most types of cancer we have treated. However, a successful regimen of metronomic low-dose chemotherapy presupposes a competent native immune system function as well.

Current immunotherapy treatment works by unleashing immune T cells from cancer-induced suppression. However, this immunological approach also presupposes a well-nourished patient with good native T-cell and other innate immune system function. If these conditions do not exist, the environment is favorable for the establishment and growth of cancer. No treatment, however well-conceived, will work well under these conditions.

The essential approach of traditional Chinese medicine, as manifested in the art of *fu zheng qu xie*, is to focus on the health of the immune system and to unswervingly keep it at the center of all treatment plans. It speaks to the same beliefs of integrative oncology practitioners that we need to support the patients physically, mentally, and spiritually before we can successfully get rid of cancer through surgery, radiation, and/or chemotherapy.

WHAT WE CAN LEARN FROM TRADITIONAL CHINESE MEDICINE

The success of Chinese doctors in treating cancer has increased since the 1960s, when the Chinese government began encouraging doctors of both Eastern and Western medicine to integrate their practice with each other. This ushered in the establishment of numerous "integrated Chinese and Western medicine hospitals" through the country.

In her book *Integrating Conventional and Chinese Medicine in Cancer Care: A Clinical Guide*,[7] Tai Lahan referred to this model as "modern Chinese medicine," which uses scientific research to validate the properties and effectiveness of Chinese herbs, formulas, and treatment regimens, such as direct intravenous administration of specially processed herbal extractions.

Clinical research conducted over several years has shown that a combined approach of integrative care using Western and Eastern medicine is more effective than employing either modality on its own. This approach has been applied more and more over the past ten years in hospital oncology departments throughout China.[8] Classical Chinese medical techniques and practices have also been integrated into Western medicine, and open-minded oncologists are using them more and more in a modern and more progressive approach to cancer treatment.

Many traditional Chinese medicine formulas have been studied by modern science methods to determine their efficacy in cancer treatment. For example, in a randomized double-blind crossover study Danshen (*Ra-*

dix salviae miltiorrhizae), a well-known Chinese herb known to have anticancer activity in traditional medicine, was found to enhance the IL-2 receptor gene expression in peripheral blood, the absolute counts of T-helper cells and CD4/CD8 T-cell ratio, and the ex-vivo production of immune-boosting Th1 cytokine profiles. The idea of using this "blood-cracking" or "blood-moving" herb to improve the cancer treatment has also been studied in research labs in China to see if it can improve the delivering of more oxygenated blood into the interior of tumors.[9] Indeed, traditional Chinese medicine—and Chinese herbs in particular—are being used to treat cancer in many ways. A few of the major uses include optimizing the effectiveness of chemotherapy or radiation by directly affecting the cancer growth, offsetting the side effects of MTD chemotherapy, enhancing the body's immunity and resistance to cancer as well as infectious disease.

Acupuncture is a discipline of traditional Chinese medicine that uses needles inserted into a patient along pressure points on meridian networks to balance *Qi* energy. Over the years it has become increasingly popular in Western countries as a support measure to control cancer-related pain, fatigue, nausea, and peripheral neuropathy from certain chemotherapy drugs. Many studies are being conducted by traditional Chinese practitioners to find more or better uses of acupuncture in oncology.

WHAT IS NATUROPATHY?

As the word *naturopathy* denotes, it is a discipline of study and practice attuned to the use of more raw and rudimentary medicine and treatment methods closely related to nature. Some elements of naturopathic medicine include food and diet as medicine, lifestyle changes, exercise plans, natural vitamins, and supplements. Naturopathy aims to support the body in a harmonious way gently and consistently, like a good life habit. It can help repair the defects and restore the balance in our physiological system to prevent or decrease cancer growth. In our own clinic, we use the toolkit of naturopathy to rein in the complications from the progression of cancer. Much of this work is the result of a close collaboration with Mark Gignac, ND, a well-known naturopathic physician in the Seattle area.

Bastyr University, a nonprofit, private university with campuses in California and Washington, is at the forefront of education, research, and practice of naturopathic medicine. According to Bastyr, naturopathic medicine is "a distinct system of primary health care that emphasizes prevention and the self-healing process through the use of natural therapies.[10] While the roots of naturopathic medicine date back to the 1890s, naturopathic medicine has witnessed a rapid increase in public interest in recent years as a result of the growing consumer movement to solve the health care puzzle, using prevention, wellness, and respect for nature's inherent healing ability."

Naturopathic practitioners dedicated to the science-based approach of naturopathic medicine observed the following six basic principles:

1. *The Healing Power of Nature (Vis Medicatrix Naturae).* Naturopathic medicine recognizes the body's inherent ability to heal itself. Naturopathic physicians identify and remove obstacles to recovery to facilitate this healing ability in patients.
2. *Identify and Treat the Causes (Tolle Causam).* The naturopathic physician seeks to identify and remove the underlying causes of illness, rather than eliminate or merely suppress symptoms.
3. *First Do No Harm (Primum Non Nocere).* Use methods and medicinal substances that minimize the risk of harmful side effects. Avoid, when possible, the harmful suppression of symptoms. Acknowledge and respect the individual's healing process, using the least force necessary to diagnose and treat illness.
4. *Doctor as Teacher (Docere).* Naturopathic physicians educate the patient and encourage self-responsibility for health. They also acknowledge the therapeutic value inherent in the doctor-patient relationship.
5. *Treat the Whole Person.* Naturopathic physicians treat each individual by taking into account physical, mental, emotional, genetic, environmental, and social factors. Since total health also includes spiritual health, naturopathic physicians encourage individuals to pursue their personal spiritual path.
6. *Prevention.* Naturopathic physicians emphasize disease prevention, assessment of risk factors, and hereditary susceptibility to disease and making appropriate interventions to prevent illness. Naturopathic medicine strives to create a healthy world in which humanity may thrive.

These principles point toward the concept of total, genuine wellness, and that is what we aim to achieve with our patients. As Bastyr states in its basic philosophy, "Wellness is a state of being healthy, characterized by positive emotion, thought, and action. Wellness is inherent in everyone, regardless of disease(s). If wellness is recognized and experienced by an individual, it will more quickly heal a given disease than direct treatment of the disease alone."

A clinical diagnosis made through the lens of naturopathy resembles traditional Chinese medicine in its focus on identifying the organic causes of disease. In the case of cancer, the focus is broader than just the tumor itself. Naturopathic therapies are drawn from research in many disciplines, including conventional medicine, European complementary medicine, clinical nutrition, botanical medicine, pharmacognosy (the branch of pharmacology dealing with the course of action, effect, and breakdown of drugs within the body), homeopathy (a medical practice based on the concept that disease can be treated with minute doses of drugs capable of producing the same symptoms as those of the disease being treated), psychology, and spirituality, as well as studies from peer-reviewed journals and clinical case studies. Therapeutic modalities used in naturopathic medicine include clinical nutrition, botanical medicine, homeopathy, physical manipulation, and acupuncture. As applied to cancer care, they integrate conventional, scientific methodology with ancient laws of nature to help find best solutions to the common cancer-related problems such as lack of energy, malnutrition, loss of appetite, nausea, constipation, insomnia, and pain. It also aims to help prevent complications from cancer treatment and to maintain or improve patient's quality of life during their treatment.

THE IMPORTANCE OF OUR MICROENVIRONMENT IN CANCER CONTROL

Understanding how cancer is affected by its surrounding environment with its interactions with immune system, and angiogenesis process, we can better grasp the importance of integrative therapies combining low-dose chemotherapy with complementary and supportive medicines. By viewing the integrative therapies under the umbrella of treatments that regulates and improves the cancer's microenvironment we can come to a better understanding of what they are, their usage, and the benefits they bring to an integrative program of cancer care.

But first what is "the microenvironment" in the context of cancer, and why is it so important that we understand it? According to the National Cancer Institute, a microenvironment refers to "the normal cells, molecules, and blood vessels that surround and feed a tumor cell. A tumor can change its microenvironment, and the microenvironment can affect how a tumor grows and spreads."

Since the war on cancer was launched decades ago, most research has been focused on cancer cell biology, with a more recent emphasis on genetics and cell-signaling mechanisms. As a result of early research, many scientists concluded that most cells, under certain conditions, could change into "immortalized" cancer cells through a specific gene-directed process.

This led to the assumption that carcinogenic agents affected cell signaling, and that their carcinogenicity was based on their effects on cancer-causing genes, or "oncogenes." Based on this theory of carcinogenesis, chemotherapeutic treatments were designed to control the cell cycle, to induce apoptosis in cancer cells, and to reduce the production of cellular signals that promote growth.

Unfortunately, these treatments have significant limitations in prolonging the lives of patients with aggressive, metastatic cancers. The fact that these treatments have met with such limited success leads to the suspicion that the underlying theory of cancer growth and control is at least incomplete. Rather than aiming treatments directly and exclusively at cancer cells and their methods of communication, we might be better off to focus the processes in the cancer's microenvironment, such as inflammation and angiogenesis, which may be essential to the progression of malignancies.

Inflammation is a central factor in every cancer development and progression, suggesting that the cellular processes occurring during inflammation are involved in the initiation of cancer. Inflammation continues to wreak havoc as the cancer grows, playing a major role throughout each and every phase of the cancer's existence, including invasion, angiogenesis, and metastasis.

Research has now shown that the invariable association of cancer and inflammation is the result of its mutagenic effects on stem cell DNA. But that's not all. Long-term behavior of tumors is significantly affected by the tumor's microenvironment. [11]

The frequent association of various tumor types with known chronic inflammatory diseases suggests that inflammation is a central factor in the biology of cancer. For example, the risk of colon cancer is associated with inflammatory bowel diseases, such as ulcerative colitis and Crohn's disease. Pancreatic cancer can be linked to pancreatitis, obesity is linked to breast cancer, gastric reflux disease may prompt esophageal cancer, and Schistosoma infections may induce bladder cancer. Research on the association of inflammation and cancer has shown that certain anti-inflammatory drugs reduce the risk of cancer development, recurrence, and metastasis, and can result in a reduction of tumor size. [12]

Angiogenesis is an important part of tumor's environment. We have referred to angiogenesis several times in this and previous chapters, and it merits a brief review. Angiogenesis refers to the formation of new blood vessels. This process involves the migration, growth, and differentiation of endothelial cells, which line the inside wall of blood vessels. [13]

The process of angiogenesis is controlled by chemical signals, such as vascular endothelial growth factors (VEGF) in the body. These signals can stimulate both the repair of damaged blood vessels and the formation of new blood vessels. Other chemical signals, called angiogenesis inhibitors, interfere with blood vessel formation. Normally, the stimulating and inhibiting effects of these chemical signals are balanced so that blood vessels form only when and where they are needed.

Angiogenesis plays a critical role in the growth and spread of cancer. A blood supply is necessary for tumors to grow beyond a few millimeters in size. Tumors can cause this blood supply to form by giving off chemical signals that stimulate angiogenesis. Tumors can also stimulate nearby normal cells to produce angiogenesis-signaling molecules. These new blood vessels feed growing tumors with oxygen and nutrients, allowing the cancer cells to invade nearby tissue, to move throughout the body, and to metastasize.

Since tumors need a blood supply to grow and/or spread, scientists are always seeking to create methods for blocking tumor angiogenesis. They study natural and synthetic angiogenesis inhibitors, focusing on how these molecules might prevent or slow the growth of cancer.

Angiogenesis requires the binding of signaling molecules, such as VEGF, to receptors on the surface of normal endothelial cells. When

VEGF and other endothelial growth factors bind to their receptors on endothelial cells, signals within these cells are initiated that promote the growth and survival of new blood vessels.

The FDA has approved several antiangiogenic drugs to treat a number of different cancers, including metastatic colorectal cancer, non-small cell lung cancers, kidney cancer, and metastatic renal cell cancer. Researchers are exploring the use of angiogenesis inhibitors to treat still other types of cancer.[14] Some commonly prescribed supplements, like curcumin, have also been shown to have significant antiangiogenesis effect.

In summary, the microenvironment of the cancer has several significant biological processes that are critical for cancer's growth and metastasis, including angiogenesis, inflammation and immune regulation. Integrative therapies aim to favorably impact all these processes to affect the cancer growth. As discussed, MLDC can provide anti-angiogenesis and immune regulation, while many integrative therapies including diet and supplement can provide synergy in reducing the inflammation, angiogenesis, and immune suppression in this setting. As an example, one of the most commonly recommended dietary supplements called curcumin has been found to have all the above beneficial effects in cancer treatments by numerous scientific studies. The benefits of taking supplements versus prescription drugs to regulate cancer's microenvironment are that dietary supplements are usually very well tolerated and can be taken on a long-term basis.

THE BENEFITS OF INTEGRATIVE MEDICINE IN SUPPORTING THE BODY'S ABILITY TO FIGHT DISEASE

As we discovered in chapter 1, MTD chemotherapy and to a lesser extent MLDC, while affecting cancer predominantly, also causes immune system problems such as decrease in immune effector cells or activity, some of which can last a long time after the treatment has been completed. Additionally, the treatments can leave some damages to various normal body structures, such as bone marrow, heart, or nerves. Some patients as a result can develop long-term problems to their health, even when their cancer is controlled or eliminated.

When physicians can utilize an expanded menu of options in treating cancer, they immediately increase their patients' chances of recovery.

Combining the best features of conventional medicine with a variety of complementary therapies is the key to increasing the odds of therapeutic success. For example, a plethora of natural medicines, including vitamins, supplements, especially different mushroom extracts, and Chinese herbs have been well documented to be either essential or beneficial in supporting the basic and specific immune functions important in cancer control.

Chinese herbs, when prescribed by a trained and experienced Chinese herbalist, can counter many side effects of chemotherapy, such as nausea, poor appetite, and myelosuppression. They build *zheng qi*, the ability of the body to increase its immunity and resistance to sickness, and also provide increased capacity to fight the cancer process independently. Moreover, Chinese herbs can potentially enhance the effectiveness of chemotherapy, allowing the patient to withstand higher or more frequent doses than they could otherwise.

This is possible because of the ability of some Chinese herbs to modify the negative side effects of chemotherapy. They do this by increasing blood cell production, by reducing the degree to which chemotherapy impairs digestive absorption, and by reducing the toxicity of chemotherapy drugs to healthy organs. When administered properly, Chinese herbs and supplements allow patients to avoid weight loss, malnourishment, extreme fatigue, and infection, thereby making a quicker and more thorough recovery possible. We do need to be aware of the potential to have negative interactions of any supplements or herbs with prescribed medications. One of the relatively well-documented interactions is the one involving St. John's Wort, a popular herb used for mild depression, and chemotherapy drugs that are metabolized through the liver's "cytochrome P450" enzyme system. St. John's Wort is known to increase the activity of this enzyme system and accelerate the degradation of the chemotherapy drug, reducing the treatment efficacy. Many herbs or supplements, such as Ginko biloba, garlic extracts, and Chinese herb Danshen can interact with warfarin and increase the risk of bleeding, Therefore, talk to an experienced natural medicine practitioner and your integrative oncologist before embarking on any new supplements or herbs.

Integrative therapy may change the relationship between a physician and his or her patients. Specifically, integrative therapy opens up opportunities for enhanced give and take, allowing doctors to focus on the health of the whole person, not just the tumor or side effect. This holistic approach to cancer care leads to better health and wellness, which should always be our overall goal.

The American Board of Physician Specialties (ABPS), the only professional body in North America offering certification in integrative medicine, emphasizes the following principles in their definition of integrative medicine:

- A close partnership between the patient and physician
- Use of both conventional and alternative medicines to treat the patient
- An emphasis on noninvasive treatments, whenever possible
- The commitment to ensuring that medical diagnoses and treatments are based on scientifically sound research
- Consideration of all factors that influence health, wellness, and disease
- An emphasis on health promotion and illness prevention through healthy living

Ideally, integrative therapy becomes a partnership between doctors and patients, instead of merely a series of prescriptions, tests, and orders. True collaboration means real listening on both sides, open discussion of treatment options, due consideration of previous experiences, and a cooperative effort in which the patient shares responsibility for his or her health by making crucial lifestyle changes.

Integrative therapy also means setting the right pace for each individual patient. This means not rushing into anything that might overwhelm the body, mind, and spirit with a tornado of drugs, testing, and treatment. Naturally, some cases require immediate attention, and the patient's immediate safety should always be the first concern. But absent a true emergency, a one-step-at-a-time approach gives the body and mind time to adjust while also providing doctors with the chance to evaluate what is working and what adjustments are in order.

The philosophy of integrative medicine is also perfect for anyone suffering from chronic issues. When, for instance, someone is dealing with constant pain, agitation, or any chronic problem, the natural approach of the integrative medicine to balance the body's different energies, such as with acupuncture and yoga exercises, can go a long way in complementing or enhancing the traditional therapies and reduce their side effects. Finally, in a health system in which patients are whisked in and out of large clinics like widgets on an assembly line, doctors practicing integrative medicine spend much more time with their patients because this is the only way to really find out who they are treating and what will work best. It also does not take a special survey to realize that patients feel better, literally and figuratively, when they are not rushed through medical processes.

INTEGRATIVE TREATMENTS WITH POTENTIAL VALUE IN CANCER TREATMENT

The list of proven integrative treatments is growing by the day. Therefore, we cannot possibly describe every treatment in sufficient detail to identify the particular set of circumstances for which a given treatment is applicable. Thus, the following list is provided mostly in an attempt to provoke further exploration on the part of interested patients and physicians, but not an endorsement or recommendations by the authors of this book.

In alphabetical order, a partial list of complementary and alternative therapies with possible values in cancer treatment or its recovery is as follows: acupressure, acupuncture, aromatherapy, art therapy, biofeedback, craniosacral therapy, counseling (individual and group), diet and nutrition, exercise and physical therapy, flower essences, hydrotherapy, hyperbaric oxygen therapy, massage, medical cannabis, meditation, melatonin, mind-body therapy, mindfulness-based stress reduction (MBSR), music therapy, ozone therapy, qi-gong, reflexology, reiki, salt rooms, tai chi, thalassotherapy, western herbal therapy, writing and journaling, and yoga.

In the following section, we provide a brief informational review of these therapies. We begin with diet and nutrition, as well as a review of several dietary supplements that have more proven value in the support of cancer treatment.

DIET AND NUTRITION

Twenty-five years ago, if you asked an MD about nutrition, he or she would either have ignored you or brushed you off with comments like "Watch your weight," or "Don't eat too many burgers." Some oncologists might have even said something to the effect of "Diet? We're dealing with cancer here! Don't worry about what you eat." The joke back then was about the "expensive urine" of "health nuts," and placebos, as if there was no science behind the contention that nutrition is vitally important to a patient's healing and overall well-being.

Fortunately, things have changed, albeit all too subtly and not so extensively as might be desired. An intelligent, motivated layperson these days can easily find abundant information with scientific notion on diet and nutrition that can play an important if not pivotal role in preventing or treating cancer.

This is a good thing, especially for patients with cancer who are receiving repeated infusions of cytotoxic chemotherapy drugs. The impact of these treatments on a person's immune system and other organs is obvious. If the body does not even have enough essential nutrients required for its normal function, how can it repair the damages and recover from the chemotherapy side effects or foster enough immune system power to fight back the cancer? For example, there are several studies over the years that many cancer patients have abnormally or even critically low vitamin C levels in their blood. However, these kinds of studies are routinely ignored by the oncology community. Some opinion leaders used the negative study results showing supplements with certain nutrients did not help with cancer prevention to conclude that nutritional supplements do not help with cancer prevention or treatment. They again fell into the trap of thinking that a single drug, in this case a vitamin, can make a difference in the outcome of a complex disease like cancer. Rather a comprehensive plan with balanced nutritional components is likely to be needed for benefiting cancer control. Looking at the success of our patients who are all on a list of complementing and balanced nutritional supplements, I have no doubt that nutritional supplements are needed and necessary for cancer patients' recovery. The value cannot be disallowed by a few pharmaceutical style studies. In the future, a more useful way of studying this issue is to compare models of care with or without imparting a comprehensive nutritional and supplement plan in their treatment.

In the following section, we will discuss general nutritional guidelines as well as more specific recommendations on particular diet programs for cancer patients.

GENERAL DIETARY GUIDELINES

According to the American Cancer Society, good nutrition is especially important if you have cancer because both the illness and its treatment can affect your appetite and amount of nutrition you can take in on a daily basis. Cancer, along with many of the treatments for it, affects the body's ability to tolerate certain foods and absorb nutrients. These problems with nutritional intake create a double jeopardy because cancer patients would actually need more nutrition than a normal person due to the increased tissue damage and repair process in their bodies. It is vital that your oncologist, or someone he or she recommends, advise you and your loved ones about your nutritional needs and help pick foods with the highest nutritional values so that you can cope with cancer and the treatment side effects.[15] For example, diarrhea, cramping, and trouble digesting food are common in the wake of the surgical removal of certain kinds of tumors. Although your doctor may recommend a low-fiber diet to reduce the severity of such a condition, it is hardly enough to really get your body on the right track nutritionally. It is also important to recognize that eating habits that are good for cancer patients can be very different from eating guidelines intended for healthy people. It is, for example, vital to remove as much sugar as possible from your diet if you are fighting cancer. There are many other changes you should make if you are a cancer patient, and they will be discussed shortly.

The National Cancer Institute defines nutrition as a process in which food is taken in and used by the body for growth, to keep the body healthy, and to replace tissue. Good health presupposes good nutrition, before, during, and after cancer and its treatment. A healthy diet includes eating and drinking enough of such essential nutrients as proteins, fats, carbohydrates, vitamins, minerals, and water. When the body does not get or cannot absorb these nutrients, it is in a condition called malnutrition or malnourishment.

In the context of cancer treatment, nutritional therapy also focuses on actions that ensure the absorption of the specific nutrients needed to restore or maintain such things as adequate body weight and strength, tissue integrity, and the prevention or treatment of infection.

As a cancer patient, you cannot afford to forget that cancer can change the way the body uses food.

Some tumors make chemicals that change the way the body uses certain nutrients. The body's use of protein, carbohydrates, and fat may be affected, especially by tumors of the gastrointestinal system. A patient may not tolerate certain food or may seem to be eating enough but not be able to absorb all the nutrients from the food.

Treatments such as surgery, chemotherapy, radiation, some types of immunotherapy, and stem cell transplantation can make it very difficult for a patient to eat well or, sometimes, at all. The same is true of cancers of the head, neck, esophagus, stomach, and intestines.

A partial list of the side effects of cancer and cancer treatment that affect eating include the following: anorexia (loss of appetite), mouth sores, dry mouth, trouble swallowing, nausea, vomiting, diarrhea, constipation, depression, anxiety, taste, and smell. Any of these issues can result in malnutrition. Malnourished patients become weak, tired, prone to infections, and unable to tolerate even mild cancer treatments. Not eating enough exacerbates the physical/mental problems further creating a vicious cycle. To break this cycle, nutritional treatment needs to focus on both fronts to mitigate problems that affect nutritional intake and provide high-value compact nutrition for the patients. In certain situations where there is no time to relieve problems associated with eating difficulties before severe malnutrition of patient will occur, such as severe inflammation/mucositis of mouth and esophagus related to radiation therapy of head and neck cancer or esophageal cancer, or small bowel obstruction due to intrabdominal cancer, temporary nutritional support in form of total parenteral nutrition (TPN), with all the essential nutrients given intravenously, needs to be considered.

Malnutrition may culminate in cachexia characterized by weight loss of over 10 percent, muscle wasting, and systemic inflammation (c-reactive protein level > 10mg/L). Cachexia often starts with weight loss but once its full spectrum is developed, the prognosis of the patient affected is very poor. To prevent/treat cachexia, one must support the patient's nutrition while treating the cancer effectively and gently.

It is important to treat weight loss caused by cancer and its treatment.

In summary, nutritional therapy should be a major element of cancer therapy whenever loss of appetite, poor digestion, constipation, nausea, vomiting, diarrhea, dry or sore mouth, persistent infections, or many different types of pain are issues.

SPECIFIC DIETARY RECOMMENDATIONS

The National Cancer Institute estimates that roughly one-third of all cancer deaths may be diet related. In this connection, it is important to remember that what you eat can hurt you, but it can also help you. Many of the common foods found in grocery stores or organic markets contain cancer-fighting properties, from the antioxidants that neutralize the damage of free radicals to the powerful phytochemicals that may fight the cancer as well as alleviate the side effects of chemotherapy. But there isn't a single element in a particular food that does all the work: the best thing to do is eat a variety of foods. [16]

According to the American Institute for Cancer Research, "No single food or food component can protect you against cancer by itself. But research shows that a diet filled with a variety of vegetables, fruits, whole grains, beans, and other plant foods help lower risk for many cancers." [17] A partial list of cancer-fighting foods includes apples, blueberries, broccoli and cruciferous vegetables, carrots, cherries, coffee, cranberries, dark green leafy vegetables, dry beans and peas, flaxseed, garlic, grapefruit, grapes and grape juice, soy, winter squash, green or black tea, tomatoes, walnuts, and whole grains. Table 4.1 below provides considerably more detail on these valuable foods that are so beneficial for cancer patients.

For dealing with a specific cancer, there may be other foods that are better suited to your diet, and I fully recommend that you find a well-versed nutritionist to help you create the diet that makes sense for your particular circumstances.

Table 4.1. Cancer-Fighting Foods and Their Modes of Action

Food	Process Affected	Details
Avocados	Muscle wasting; general anticancer compounds	Rich in glutathione; reduces free radicals by blocking absorption of certain fats; more potassium than bananas; good source of beta-carotene, which suppresses lung, mouth, throat, stomach, intestine, bladder, prostate, and breast cancer.
Carrots	General anticancer compounds	Rich in beta carotene and falcarinol (raw carrots), both of which are anticancer compounds.[1]
Cruciferous vegetables (broccoli, brussels sprouts, cabbage, cauliflower, and kale)	Antiestrogen (breast cancer); anticancer compounds (colorectal, prostate)	Contains indole-3-carbinol, which converts cancer-promoting estrogen into a more protective form; sulforaphane (especially sprouts), which helps prevent colorectal cancer[2]; and lutein and zeaxanthin, antioxidants that fight prostate cancer. Kale also contains isothiocyanates, phytochemicals that suppress tumor growth and block carcinogens from reaching their targets.
Chili peppers	Anticancer compounds (stomach)	Contain capsaicin, which may neutralize certain cancer-causing nitrosamines and thereby help prevent stomach cancer.
Citrus fruits	Carcinogen removal	Contain monoterpenes, which help prevent cancer by removing carcinogens. Oranges and lemons contain limonene, which stimulates cancer-killing lymphocytes that may also break down cancer-causing substances.

Food	Process Affected	Details
Figs	Shrinks tumors	Contain a derivative of benzaldehyde, which shrinks tumors; also vitamins A and C, and calcium, magnesium, and potassium.[3]
Flax	Anticancer compounds (colon; general)	Contains lignans, which are antioxidants that block or suppress cancer; also omega-3 fatty acids, which protect against colon cancer.
Garlic	Immune enhancement; carcinogen deactivation; anticancer effects (stomach, colon)	Contains immune-enhancing allium compounds that also break down cancer-causing substances in the liver, block carcinogens from entering cells, and slow tumor development. Studies show garlic, onions, leeks, and chives lower risk of stomach and colon cancer.[4] People who consume raw or cooked garlic regularly face about half the risk of stomach cancer and two-thirds the risk of colorectal cancer as people who eat little or none.[5]
Grapes	Inhibit growth of cancer cells; release immune system from suppression	Contain bioflavonoids, resveratrol and ellagic acid. Bioflavonoids are anticancer antioxidants; resveratrol inhibits growth-promoting enzymes that stimulate growth of cancer cells and suppress the immune response; and ellagic acid also blocks enzymes that promote tumor growth.
Licorice root	Anticancer compounds (prostate)	Contains glycyrrhizin, which blocks a component of testosterone and may help prevent the growth of prostate cancer.

Food	Process Affected	Details
Nuts	Inhibit growth of cancer cells; anticancer compounds (prostate)	Contain the antioxidants quercetin and campferol, which suppress cancer growth. Brazil nuts contain 80 micrograms of selenium, important to controlling prostate cancer (patient with nut allergies should take selenium supplements instead).
Papayas	Reduce absorption of carcinogens	Contain the antioxidant vitamin C, which reduces the absorption of nitrosamines, as well as folic acid, which minimizes the effects of certain cancers.
Raspberries	General nutrition; anticancer compounds (colon, pancreatic)	Contain many vitamins, minerals, phytochemicals, and anticancer antioxidants known as anthocyanins. Black raspberries, richer in antioxidants than strawberries or blueberries, fight both colon and pancreatic cancer.
Red wine	General anticancer compounds; cell division inhibitor	Contains polyphenols, potent antioxidants that protect against various cancers by neutralizing free radicals. Also contains resveratrol, which inhibits cell proliferation and can help to prevent cancer. Nonalcoholic wine may be medically preferable.
Seaweed and other sea vegetables	Anticancer compounds (lung, mouth, throat, stomach, intestine, bladder, prostate, and breast cancer); general nutrition	Contain beta-carotene, protein, vitamin B12, fiber, and chlorophyll, as well as chlorophylones, important fatty acids that fight against breast cancer. Sea vegetables also are rich in potassium, calcium, magnesium, iron, and iodine.

Food	Process Affected	Details
Soy products	Antiangiogenic; suppresses growth of epithelial cells; anticancer compounds (breast)	Contain phytoestrogenic isoflavones that depress breast cancer by both hormonal and nonhormonal processes. Also contain genistein, a potent inhibitor cancer growth and spread that works by inhibiting the growth of epithelial cells and new blood vessels for growing tumors. Patients should, however, limit soy consumption lest hormone imbalances stimulate cancer growth. Women with or at risk of breast cancer should talk to their doctors before taking pure soy isoflavone powder or pills.
Sweet potatoes	Antimutagenic	Contain many anticancer properties, including beta-carotene, which protects DNA in the cell nucleus from cancer-causing chemicals outside the nuclear membrane.
Teas, black and green	Prevent cancer cell division	Contain polyphenol antioxidants (catechins) that prevent cancer cells from dividing. Green tea is best, followed by the more common black tea. Herbal teas, however, do not have these benefits.

Food	Process Affected	Details
Tomatoes	Anticancer compounds (breast, prostate, pancreas, and colorectal cancer)	Contain lycopene, an antioxidant that reduces oxygen free radicals suspected of triggering cancer. It appears that the hotter the weather, the more lycopene tomatoes produce. Watermelons, carrots, and red peppers also contain lycopene in lesser quantities. Lycopene is concentrated when tomatoes are cooked. Increased lycopene consumption reduces risk of breast, prostate, pancreas, and colorectal cancer.
Turmeric	Anticancer compounds (breast, prostate, pancreas, and colorectal cancer)	A member of the ginger family, it inhibits production of the inflammation-related enzyme cyclo-oxygenase 2 (COX-2), whose levels are abnormally high in certain inflammatory diseases and cancers, especially bowel and colon cancer.

THE KETOGENIC DIET

At its core, a ketogenic diet deprives cancer cells of their sources of energy—glucose. It consists mainly of fat intake (90 percent), with a small amount of protein (8 percent), and very little carbohydrates (2 percent). Some examples of good fat may come from avocados, coconut oil, olive oil, raw seeds, nuts, and fatty fish like salmon. Protein sources may come from fish, egg, organic grass-fed beef, poultry, fermented dairy, and grass-fed dairy. Low-carb food may come from some veggies, like cauliflower, cabbage, spinach, asparagus, collard greens, and kales. These proportions force the body to burn fat instead of glucose through the oxidation of fatty acids in the liver to produce ketone bodies, which can be used by normal cells, such as brain or muscle cells, but not cancer cells, to produce energy.

Ketogenic diets show promise because they exploit inherent oxidative metabolic differences between cancer cells and normal cells. In simpler terms, a ketogenic diet might have therapeutic effects because cancer cells "feed on" glucose. It's estimated that cancer cells have ten times the ability of normal cells to concentrate glucose but only 1/10 efficiency to utilize glucose in energy production through a biochemical process called glycolysis. This leads to accumulation of lactic acid in cancer cells, which cancer cells can recycle to produce more energy. The metabolism of glucose by cancer cells also creates more inflammation and tissue acidification making cancer cells more resistant to chemotherapy treatment. Unlike normal cells, cancer cells are unable to metabolize the ketone bodies derived from the fats that are mobilized by the ketogenic diet. Thus, in general terms, a ketogenic diet has the potential to starve cancer cells.

Although the entire spectrum of anticancer impacts attributable to a ketogenic diet when combined with standard radiation or chemotherapy is not yet known, preclinical trials of the diet combined with radiation and/ or chemotherapy have shown positive responses in mouse cancer models and anecdotal cases of prolonged cancer control using ketogenic diet alone in human patients have been reported.

Low carbohydrate diets have been studied as an adjuvant to cancer therapy in both animal models and case studies of human patients. Researchers at the CRC Experimental Chemotherapy Group observed decreased tumor weight and reduced cachexia in mice with colon adenocarcinoma xenografts eating a ketogenic diet. Additional studies have shown that ketogenic diets reduce tumor growth and improve survival in animal models of malignant glioma, colon cancer, gastric cancer, and prostate cancer.[18]

Researchers have also found promise in using ketogenic diets to temper the effects of radiation in malignant glioma models and in treating non-small cell lung cancer.

Fasting, which induces a state of ketosis, has been found to enhance responsiveness to chemotherapy in preclinical cancer therapy animal models and may reduce some of the normal tissue side effects seen with chemotherapy. Fasting cycles have also been found to slow the growth of tumors. There is, therefore, some reason to think a brief fast before undergoing chemotherapy may increase the impact on cancer cells.

A recent study exploring quality of life of human patients with advanced cancer discovered that when these patients adopted a ketogenic diet, their emotional state improved and they slept better, while experiencing no negative effects. There may, however, be some potential negative consequences to such a high fat content in the diet. These negative effects include lethargy, nausea, vomiting, and a substantial increase in cholesterol. Previous studies also reveal deficiencies in trace minerals, such as selenium, copper, and zinc, which may be counteracted by dietary supplementation.

Eleven trials currently under way are assessing low carbohydrate diets as an adjuvant cancer therapy. One, conducted at the University of Würzburg in Germany, involved patients who had found no success with traditional cancer therapy and had run out of options. These patients were enrolled in trials involving the ketogenic diet. Preliminary reports show that those who continued the ketogenic diet for more than three months showed an improvement and stabilization in their physical condition, as well as shrinking or slowed growth in their tumors.[19] Another German study designed to determine whether a mild ketogenic diet could influence quality of life and survival for patients with recurrent glioblastoma found that the diet had no severe adverse effects.[20] Similar phase 1 trials at the University of Iowa are assessing the tolerability of a ketogenic diet in combination with chemotherapy and radiation therapy for patients with locally advanced pancreas, lung, and head and neck cancer.[21]

DIETARY SUPPLEMENTS

From vitamins, minerals, and herbs, to products made from plants, animal parts, algae, seafood, and yeast, the world of dietary supplements is large enough to be overwhelming. There is also an endless amount of controversy surrounding what supplements should be avoided, which ones should be used, and how they should be used most effectively. This proper use varies from patient to patient, depending on a number of factors that should be discussed with your medical team. We describe here some supplements that have proven to be effective in our practice with a multitude of cancer patients.

IMMUNE-BOOSTING EFFECTS OF MUSHROOM EXTRACTS

Mushrooms have a long history of medicinal use in many Asian countries. While they have only recently gained notice and popularity in Western countries, several studies demonstrate that the active biological compounds found in naturally growing mushrooms have a great deal of promise in treating cancer. One of the anticancer substances found in mushrooms include compounds called beta-glucans, which keep immune cells alert. Another is ergothioneine, a strong antioxidant that helps lower inflammation throughout the body.

Traditional Chinese medicine uses more than two hundred species of mushrooms to treat a variety of ailments, and approximately 25 percent of the mushrooms used have been found to contain anticancer compounds that can help fight cancerous tumors more effectively. They can do this by inhibiting tumor cell aggregation and formation and cell mutation. At the same time, mushroom extracts protect healthy cells and increase the body's inner power to destroy cancer cells.

According to a review by the medical journal *Biotech*, mushrooms as "anti-cancer compounds play a crucial role as a reactive oxygen species inducer, mitotic kinase inhibitor, anti-mitotic, and angiogenesis inhibitor, which lead to stop of cancer proliferation . . . and eventually cancer cell apoptosis."[22] They are also one of the best foods available for increasing natural killer (NK) cells, the type of immune cells that seek out and destroy dangerous cancerous cells.

According to a 2005 report published in the *Journal of Evidence-Based Complementary and Alternative Medicine*, mushrooms contain "compounds and complex substances with antimicrobial, antiviral, antitumor, antiallergic, immunomodulating, anti-inflammatory, antiatherogenic, hypoglycemic, and hepatoprotective activities."[23] While this technical jargon may take some time to digest, the take-home message is that mushrooms protect us from bacteria and viruses, attack tumors, enhance the immune system, reduce atherosclerosis, reduce the preferred food of cancer cells, protect the blood forming tissue, and reduce inflammation, the root cause of most disease. They do this by bolstering many systems in the body, and they can also help to make the body more alkaline. It has been shown that cancer cells are unable to grow in an alkaline environment.[24]

Another mushroom extract known as Active Hexose Correlated Compound (AHCC) is one of the leading supplements used in Japan to enhance the immune system. Japanese researchers, in conjunction with the Yale School of Medicine, found that AHCC also reduces the growth rate of cancer cells by increasing the production of cytokines by white blood cells. AHCC has also been found to reduce the side effects of chemotherapy.[25] Mushrooms found to have positive anticancer effects include shiitakes, cordyceps, enoki, maitake, reishi, Lion's Mane, and Turkey Tail. Using them in extract form is the best way to create optimal effects in cancer treatment.

ANTI-INFLAMMATORY EFFECTS OF CURCUMIN

Curcumin (diferuloylmethane) is the phytochemical component found in turmeric, which has been used in India for centuries as a dietary spice and a topical ointment for the treatment of inflammation. It is relatively insoluble in water, but dissolves in acetone, dimethylsulphoxide, and ethanol. Turmeric is a perennial herb that is part of the ginger family and generally grows in southeast tropical Asia. The root of this plant, the rhizome, which has been widely used in traditional Indian Ayurvedic medicine to treat a variety of issues, and ancient Indian medical texts describe using curcumin to treat inflammatory diseases, wound healing, and abdominal problems. In fact, today we can see a lower incidence of colon cancer among Indians who regularly use turmeric in their traditional cooking.

Some in today's scientific community have seen the anticancer effects of curcumin in its ability to block initiation, promotion, invasion, angiogenesis, and metastasis. It has also been shown to modulate angiogenesis, which when uncontrolled can promote tumor growth and metastasis. In addition to these effects, curcumin has a very important role as an anti-inflammatory agent.

A limited number of studies on cancer patients have examined the pharmacokinetic properties of curcumin. In one phase I study of fifteen patients with advanced colorectal cancer, six patients were given 3.6 grams of curcumin daily for up to four months. This daily dosing resulted in a detectable level of curcumin and its conjugates in plasma. Urine samples from these patients showed 0.1 to $1.3 \mu M$ curcumin and trace levels of its conjugates. Since curcumin can be detected in the urine samples, urine analysis can be used as a measure of general compliance and to assess inter- and intra-individual variability.[26]

Along with the dose studies, malignant colorectal tissues were analyzed in patients consuming 3.6 grams of curcumin daily for seven days prior to surgery. The concentrations of curcumin in normal and malignant colorectal tissues of patients were 12.7 ± 5.7 and 7.7 ± 1.8nmol/g. Curcumin conjugates were seen in the intestinal tissue of these patients and trace levels of curcumin were found in peripheral circulation. A daily oral dose of 3.6 grams of curcumin resulted in a pharmacologically efficacious level in colorectal tissues. Further studies may prove benefits with different types of cancer, too.

Based on a number of clinical studies in carcinogenesis, a daily oral dose of 3.6 grams of curcumin has been shown to be potentially effective for preventing colorectal cancer development, with curcumin functioning as an anti-inflammatory agent contributes to the upregulation of peroxisome proliferator-activated receptor-γ (PPAR-γ) activation.[27] Numerous studies have also shown the importance of curcumin as a potent immunomodulatory agent in T cells, B cells, neutrophils, natural killer cells, dendritic cells, and macrophages.[28]

In summary, curcumin is a well-tolerated, potent anti-inflammatory with demonstrated abilities to reduce the incidence of colorectal cancer and possibly other cancers. Its anticancer effects are attributable to its ability to reduce inflammation, to activate the adaptive immune system and to suppress the vascularization of tumors. Moreover, it has been shown to possess these abilities by infiltrating into living tumors when consumed in relatively low doses.

ANTI-INFLAMMATORY EFFECTS OF GREEN TEA EXTRACT

While green tea has been a staple for people all over the world for thousands of years, consumed as a drink, in edible form, and as an extract, scientists have only recognized it for its medicinal benefits over the past few decades. The antioxidants in green tea have potent anti-inflammatory qualities, and this has led to its use in treating diseases caused by inflammation, including atherosclerosis, liver disease, inflammatory bowel disease, and a variety of cancers.

According to the National Cancer Institute (NCI), a 2012 cancer prevention research conference presented evidence that men with prostate cancer who consumed green tea before undergoing prostate removal surgery had reduced inflammation markers. The NCI also noted that men with a specific precursor to prostate cancer reduced their risk of developing the disease by consuming green tea.[29] The University of Maryland Medical Center has reported that green tea has positive effects in treating a variety of other cancers, including prostate, stomach, skin, pancreatic, ovarian, breast, lung, esophageal, and colorectal.[30]

Epigallocatechin gallate (EGCG) is the active ingredient of green tea. A 2011 study published in *Lasers in Surgery and Medicine* found that the anti-inflammatory properties of EGCG increased cancer cell death in breast cancer cells.[31] Another study showed that EGCG may eliminate tumor cells when used in conjunction with chemotherapy or radiation. Moreover, a series of reports since 2002 showed that EGCG has anti-inflammatory effects.

It is known that specific genes code for the inflammatory cytokine interleukin-8. When researchers isolated this gene in a laboratory to see what effect EGCG would have, they found that the more EGCG they applied to the gene, the less capable it was of producing the effects that normally lead to inflammation. Other studies confirming these findings emphasized that when EGCG is more concentrated, as it is in whole green tea leaves and in extract form, it is even more effective.

ANTI-INFLAMMATORY EFFECTS OF FISH OIL

The wide-ranging health benefits of fish oil and omega-3 fatty acids in general are now widely known. Pharmaceutical companies have paid close attention to these trends and, with adequate science at their back, have come up with many relatively inexpensive prescription fish oils. But when it comes to protecting yourself against disease and the aging process, these costly products are not necessary, especially because most everyone now has access to over-the-counter fish oil supplements. That being said, it is important to make sure you are purchasing a quality version of what your doctor recommends.

A landmark study at the University of California, San Diego, in 2012 found that components in fish oil deters inflammation from developing in the body and also diminishes inflammation that already exists. While previous studies showed the wide range of health benefits of omega-3s, scientists are still discovering exactly how they function in the body and produce their results.[32]

Recent reports in Harvard Health Publications and other medical periodicals[33] raise questions about how much fish oil is safe to consume, as some research indicates too much can increase the risk of prostate cancer. While it is obviously very important to be vigilant about unsafe supplements, we have seen good results in many patients when fish oil was added to their regimen of supplements.

THE SPECIAL BENEFITS OF USING HIGH-DOSE INTRAVENOUS VITAMIN C

Another vital element of a naturopathic regimen is fighting cancer with bio-oxidation by administering high doses of vitamin C intravenously. Unfortunately, there are many misconceptions regarding vitamin C and cancer in the world of oncology at this time. I would like to take some time to dispel some of this confusion and to describe the many benefits of high-dose IV vitamin C by presenting several case studies which validate its use.

Vitamin C (ascorbic acid) is an essential nutrient found in food and dietary supplements that the body cannot produce on its own. According to the National Cancer Institute, vitamin C is considered an antioxidant that helps prevent oxidative stress and cell damage by free radicals. It also works with enzymes to produce collagen, the most abundant protein in the body and the substance that literally holds us together.

Vitamin C is found in all fruits and vegetables, especially citrus fruits, strawberries, cantaloupe, green peppers, tomatoes, broccoli, leafy greens, and potatoes. It is water soluble and must be taken every day.

It is important to note that vitamin C can reach much higher concentrations in the blood when taken intravenously than orally.

Since early research was conducted in the 1970s, high-dose vitamin C has been studied as a treatment for patients with cancer. Ewan Cameron, a Scottish surgeon, worked with Nobel Prize–winning chemist Linus Pauling to study the possible benefits of vitamin C therapy in clinical trials of cancer patients in the late 1970s and early 1980s. It was proposed at the time that high-dose ascorbic acid could help build resistance to disease or infection, and possibly treat cancer.[34]

Subsequent studies have shown that high doses of vitamin C can indeed slow the growth and spread of prostate, pancreatic, liver, colon, and other types of cancer, as well as improve physical, mental, and emotional functioning, symptoms of fatigue, nausea, vomiting, pain, and loss of appetite.[35]

Based on the work of several research pioneers, high-dose IV vitamin C has been proven to be selectively toxic to cancer cells if given intravenously. Research published by Dr. Mark Levine at the National Institutes of Health confirmed that vitamin C, when administered intravenously, serves as a nontoxic chemotherapeutic agent that can be given in conjunction with chemotherapy.[36]

Vitamin C interacts with iron and other metals to create hydrogen peroxide. In high concentrations, hydrogen peroxide damages the DNA and mitochondria of cancer cells, closes down their energy supply, and destroys them. And, perhaps most importantly, vitamin C has not been found to be toxic to healthy normal cells—unlike chemotherapy drugs—even at very high doses. This supports the doctor's oath of "First Do No Harm." One exception is for patients with inherited genetic deficiency in "G6PD" enzyme, in which case vitamin C can induce severe red blood cell hemolysis. Although this condition is very rare, it is still a good idea to check the blood G6PD enzyme level before giving high-dose intravenous vitamin C.

As mentioned, studies have shown that high-dose intravenous vitamin C can be effective against many types of cancer, including lung, brain, colon, breast, pancreatic, and ovarian cancer. Some studies found that when human cancers are grafted into animals, high-dose IV vitamin C decreases tumor size by 41 percent to 53 percent in diverse cancer types known for both their aggressive growth and limited treatment options.[37]

Regarding colorectal cancer, high-dose IV vitamin C impairs the growth of both KRAS and BRAF gene-mutated colorectal tumors. When vitamin C enters malignant cells, it triggers an attack entailing so much oxidative stress that the cells "burn out" and die. It is interesting that the anticancer effect of vitamin C depends on a degree of seeming duplicity. Vitamin C does not enter cancer cells as vitamin C, but as another substance known as dehydroascorbic acid, or DHA. Cancer cells are "duped" into ingesting the DHA, which quickly reverts to ascorbic acid once inside. Then, as mentioned, a series of chemical reactions characteristic of cancer cells results in the conversion of ascorbic acid to lethal concentrations of hydrogen peroxide.

These findings confirm Linus Pauling's speculation about the benefits of intravenous vitamin C as a cancer therapy. Clearly, high-dose IV vitamin C presents new possibilities of increasing the survival of cancer patients above levels attainable by conventional chemotherapy only.

Since the body needs high levels of vitamin C to achieve these results, oral ingestion is not sufficient. This is likely why early studies by Mayo Clinic researchers from the 1970s did not find benefits in cancer control in patients taking relatively large doses of oral vitamin C. Intravenous vitamin C administration is preferable because it bypasses normal digestive processes that include the production of hydrogen peroxide in tissues that are equipped to process hydrogen peroxide into nonlethal substances. Cancer cells have no such ability. Moreover, the leakage of hydrogen peroxide from disintegrating cancer cells enhances the disease-fighting abilities of white blood cells, with further anticancer impacts.

Although high-dose intravenous ascorbic acid has caused very few side effects in clinical trials, it is not patentable and therefore has not been submitted to the U.S. Food and Drug Administration by any pharmaceutical companies for approval in the treatment for cancer. However, just based on the studies that show that a large proportion of cancer patients are critically deficient in blood vitamin C level, it is worthwhile to give cancer patients some vitamin C. As discussed in the next chapter, we have seen extensive benefits to intravenously administered vitamin C in the adjunctive treatment of many different cancer patients in our practice.

GLUTATHIONE AND L-GLUTAMINE

Glutathione is composed of three simple amino acids—cysteine, glycine, and glutamine. It is a major antioxidant and a vital component of our defense system. Like other antioxidants, it protects tissues from free radicals by detoxifying active species and/or the repair of injury. It also plays a critical role in the metabolism of drugs and, when transformed into one of the enzymes called glutathione-S-transferases, the detoxification of xenobiotic (substances not normally present) toxins.[38]

Low levels of glutathione are associated with immune deficiency, progression of chronic diseases, and aging. Along with antioxidant defense of the cell, glutathione plays a central role in drug detoxification and the cellular communication that is necessary to regulate gene expression, cell death, and cell growth.

Studies also suggest that intravenous glutathione reduces toxicity and cancer side effects, improves or maintains quality of life, and enhances therapeutic effects in some cancer patients treated with certain chemotherapy agents.[39] A randomized double-blind placebo-controlled study of glutathione in combination with oxaliplatin-based chemotherapy demonstrated significant reduction of chemo-induced sensory neuropathy without clinical reduction of oxaliplatin efficacy. Glutathione may also help treat cancer cachexia. The progression of cancer cachexia is associated with the depletion of intracellular glutathione and with increases in markers of oxidative stress due to high levels of toxicity in the body.[40] Some research indicates glutathione should not be administered with antioxidant chemotherapy agents because of interference.[41]

L-glutamine is a nonessential branched-chain amino acid. It is an important nontoxic nitrogen carrier in the body and an important constituent of dairy products, fish, and green leafy vegetables. It participates in a variety of physiological functions and is a major fuel source for enterocytes (absorptive cells in the small intestine) and a substrate for gluconeogenesis in the kidney, lymphocytes, and monocytes. It is also a major component of muscle protein and is often administered in the wake of infection, inflammation, and muscle trauma.[42]

Cancer produces a state of L-glutamine deficiency, which is further aggravated by toxic effects of chemotherapeutic agents. L-glutamine deficiency increases the tolerance of tumors to chemotherapy, and reduces the tolerance of normal tissues to the side effects of chemotherapy. Although current data supports the usefulness of L-glutamine supplementation in reducing complications of chemotherapy, the paucity of explicit clinical trials weakens a clear interpretation of this general finding.

States of physiologic stress, including those resulting from the treatment of malignant disease, are characterized by a relative deficiency of L-glutamine. Supplementation with this inexpensive dietary supplement may have an important role in the prevention of gastrointestinal, neurologic, and, possibly, cardiac complications of cancer therapy. These complications often severely degrade quality of life, and may also force changes to less effective therapies. L-glutamine may also improve the therapeutic index of both chemotherapy and radiation. Two of the main uses of L-glutamine supplementation during chemotherapy, as supported by clinical studies, are prevention of chemotherapy-induced mucositis and peripheral neuropathy, particularly that related to chemotherapy drugs oxaliplatin and Taxol.

Although it is well known that cancer cells under certain circumstances, do ingest L-glutamine for energy, no human studies have shown that L-glutamine increases tumor growth. Over the last twenty years, thirty-six clinical trials have demonstrated the benefits of L-glutamine supplementation in cancer patients with improvement of their metabolism and clinical situation without increasing tumor growth. In our own experience, nearly all our patients on either Taxol or oxaliplatin treatments over the last twenty years have been recommended to take L-glutamine 10 to 15 grams twice a day to help prevent neuropathy and the highly consistent tumor responses we have seen in these patients defuses any concern one may have regarding the safety of L-glutamine supplementation during chemotherapy treatments.

INTEGRATIVE TREATMENTS FROM A TO Z

Here we offer a large menu of possible therapies, ranging from those that address specific physical and medical issues to those related to your emotional, psychological, and spiritual needs. Based on their needs and special interests, patients may select from this list one or a few of the complementary therapies to help them through the cancer journey.

Acupressure

This ancient Asian technique is similar to acupuncture, but does not use needles. Practitioners use their hands or tools to apply pressure to various acupoints on the body to open energy flows, release tension, and promote emotional balance. Stimulating various points on the body can trigger the release of endorphins, the body's pain-reducing chemicals, and increase the flow of blood and oxygen to areas of the body to relieve discomfort and soreness. Acupressure is often used to treat chronic muscle or joint pain, headache, and to induce relaxation.

Acupuncture

A key component of traditional Chinese medicine, acupuncture is practiced by inserting extremely thin needles through the skin at strategic acupoints on your body. The goal is to rebalance the flow of energy or life force within the body, which is known as *Qi*.

Acupuncture needles are so thin that most people feel little to no pain.

The needles stimulate acupoints, which cause the nervous system to release opium-like endorphins to the muscles, spinal cord, and brain. This can reduce the experience of pain and trigger the release of other chemicals and hormones that influence the body's internal regulating system.

There are a few conditions for which sound research has demonstrated acupuncture therapy to be an effective and safe adjunct therapy for cancer care. Randomized clinical trials have shown that acupuncture can significantly reduce the development and severity of chemotherapy-induced nausea and vomiting. Other researches have also suggested its benefits in managing cancer-related pain, cancer fatigue, chemotherapy-induced neutropenia, and radiation-induced xerostomia.

Aromatherapy

Aromatic essential oils from plants are extracted, distilled, and typically mixed with other substances, such as alcohol or lotion. They are then applied to the skin, sprayed into the air, or inhaled. Inhaling a scent triggers powerful neurotransmitters and other chemicals that stimulate certain parts of the limbic system, which control emotions and behavior, resulting in an improved mood. Aromatherapy is used to treat stress, sleep disorders, and mood disturbances, including depression and anxiety.

Art therapy

Many visual creations, especially those done directly by a patient, cause a powerful, positive impact on a person's psyche. These impacts can translate into positive effects on the body as well. This type of self-expression can influence physical, emotional, cognitive, and social well-being. Art therapy is used to treat all kinds of people facing difficult health challenges, including cancers.

Biofeedback

This treatment technique trains people to improve their health using signals from their own bodies. Sensors are attached to your body to provide instant feedback on things like heart rate, blood pressure, skin temperature, and muscle tension. After reviewing the results on a monitor, the biofeedback therapist then teaches you mental and physical exercises to control those functions. Biofeedback is used to treat urinary incontinence, stress, anxiety, and depression that may be associated with advanced cancer.

Craniosacral therapy

More than a hundred years ago, an osteopath discovered that cranial bones are related to tissues and fluids in the body and its central nervous system. This gentle form of massage therapy, used by chiropractors, massage therapists, and naturopaths, involves finger pressure to manipulate the bones of the skull, lower spine, and pelvis.

Some believe that the craniosacral system, consisting of membranes and fluids that surround and protect the brain and spinal cord, has a rhythm that is felt throughout the body and influences the functioning of the central nervous system. Using a very light touch, skilled practitioners can pinpoint sources of stress and help the body self-correct by assisting in the natural movement of the fluid and related soft tissue. Craniosacral therapy is used to treat back pain, headaches, and other problems triggered within the nervous system.

Counseling (individual and group)

A diagnosis of cancer creates multiple issues, some of which require the expertise of an oncology social worker. This person is a licensed professional who provides emotional support while helping people access practical assistance, through services such as individual counseling, support groups, services for home care or facility transportation, and even securing disability payments or other forms of financial assistance. Continuous individual counseling may be used to treat a range of emotional issues, including the sense of isolation, depression, guilt, and alienation of family relationships during cancer treatment. Additional teaching of coping skills such as meditation and guided imagery are also often provided.

Exercise

A study from American Cancer Society shows that regular exercise is associated with lower risk of thirteen specific subtypes of cancer. It has also been linked to reduced fatigue and physical endurance of cancer patients during chemotherapy. A mild and moderate aerobic exercise program can be prescribed as a treatment for fatigue related to cancer. Importantly, a systemic Medline review of evidence found that patients diagnosed with cancer demonstrated a trend toward increased survival with greater level of physical activity. In a study on 933 patients with local regional breast cancer, any moderate-intensity exercise after diagnosis reduced mortality risk by 64 percent compared to an inactive woman. Similar findings were demonstrated in patients with colorectal cancer. Animal studies appear to show that exercise decreases inflammatory signaling in the tumor microenvironment, thereby decreasing tumor angiogenesis. The American Society of Clinical Oncology (ASCO) recommend cancer survivors meet the recommended 2.5 hours per week of moderate exercise to the extent their physical condition allows.

Flower essences

Dr. Edward Bach created the flower essence system in the 1930s. He believed that distilled essences of wildflowers, usually preserved in an alcohol base and administered internally, under the tongue, could help heal emotional disturbances.[43]

Flower essence therapy is considered "vibrational medicine," based on the idea that everything in nature, including flowers and your own body, has its own vibration. When a vibration is out of tune in the body, which can be caused by emotional distress and illness, using flower essences with its own specific vibration can help restore a sense of calm and balance. Flower essences are used to treat stress, bad moods, and flagging energy levels.

Hydrotherapy

The healing power of water is used to treat disease or maintain optimal health. Hydrotherapy takes various forms, including steam or mineral baths, saunas, hot or cold wet body wraps, aquatic physical therapy, and whirlpools. Practitioners say that immersion treatments and wraps detoxify the blood, enhance the immune system, and expand blood vessels. Native Americans traditionally used sweat lodges as a type of remedy to cleanse poisons from the body. Hydrotherapy is used to treat pain, atopic dermatitis, psoriasis, and knee osteoarthritis.

Hyperbaric oxygen therapy

Hyperbaric oxygen chambers with pressurized pure oxygen from 1.5 to 3 atmosphere levels have mainly been used to help heal chronic skin wounds such as those of burn victims. It may thus also be helpful in healing of wounds related to cancer or its treatment. Since studies have shown that it may increase the oxygen level in the hypoxic tumor tissues, it may increase the sensitivity of tumor cells to chemo or radiotherapy by inducing oxidative stress. It's generally safe to be used as an adjunctive cancer therapy but more studies are needed to demonstrate its value as a cancer treatment. Subjectively, patients going through this therapy have reported better energy level, possibly due to improved oxygenation of the blood.

Massage

Using the principle that touch is healing, massage involves rubbing the soft tissues of the body, such as the muscles and connective tissues, to release tension or treat injury. There are over eighty different types of massage. Some are gentle, such as Swedish massage, and others are very active, such as Thai massage, or intense, such as deep tissue massage.

Aside from creating an ultimate sense of relaxation, massage works on the cellular level to reduce inflammation and promote the growth of new mitochondria in skeletal muscle, stimulating the healing of connective tissues or damaged muscles. Massage is used to treat migraines, improve sleep quality, enhance immune function, and reduce lower back pain.

Medical cannabis

Medical cannabis, also known as marijuana, refers to any part of the marijuana plant that may be used to treat health problems. These plants contain many chemicals, known as cannabinoids. Two main cannabinoids are THC and CBD. THC provides some of the pleasurable effects that people seek, but it also has some effects that may treat medical problems. Some research suggests that CBD may be helpful for some health issues as well, but CBD doesn't cause you to get high. For that reason, some people use medical cannabis that only contains CBD. Studies spanning more than three decades have shown that medical marijuana is an effective treatment for some symptoms of cancer as well as the side effects of chemotherapy and radiation therapy, from nausea and vomiting to loss of appetite, fatigue, insomnia, and anxiety. THC, in particular, has been shown to decrease cancer-related pain. Additionally, numerous preclinical studies have demonstrated that both THC and CBD possess anticancer cell activity. However, it's still unclear whether similar levels of cannabis can be achieved inside patient's body safely to have the same cancer-killing effects.

Meditation

This ancient practice is a simple and relatively easy way to reduce stress on the mind and body by refocusing attention on calming thoughts and/or the breath. Meditation takes many forms, including mindfulness meditation, repeating a mantra, guided imagery, or visualization.

By reducing the activity of the sympathetic nervous system, which is responsible for the anxiety-inducing "fight or flight" response, meditation can lower your heart rate, slow your breathing, lower your blood pressure, and relax your muscles. Meditation also changes the structure of the cerebral cortex in the brain, which plays an instrumental role in memory, attention, thought, and consciousness. Researches on mindfulness-based stress reduction (MBSR) have shown that MBSR can help relieve particular symptoms and improve quality of life of cancer patients. Interestingly, a researcher from Canada recently found that support groups that encouraged meditation and yoga can alter the cellular activity of cancer survivors. Meditation is used to treat anxiety, stress, chronic pain, and depression in cancer patients.

Melatonin

Melatonin is a hormone produced naturally by the pineal gland. This occurs in response to darkness. Levels remain high during sleep until the pineal gland, responding to light, turns off production. Since its discovery in the 1950s, the effect melatonin has on cancer has been a subject of study. In the mid-1990s, a form of synthetic melatonin became available as a nutritional supplement, largely aimed at helping people with a variety of sleep issues.

Melatonin also has immune-boosting effects. As far as cancer is concerned, melatonin levels are important to monitor. According to a University of Maryland Medical Center study, women with breast cancer typically have lower levels of melatonin than women who don't. Similarly, men with prostate cancer typically have lower melatonin levels than other men.[44] The American Cancer Society has reported that some studies show shift workers with irregular sleep schedules have an increased risk of cancer. Beyond the normal aging process, melatonin levels can be lowered by caffeine, alcohol, and tobacco consumption. When it comes to the immune system and cancer, melatonin may play a significant role because of its antioxidant effects and its ability to stimulate the immune system to attack cancer cells.

A review of melatonin in the treatment of solid tumors by randomized controlled trials and meta-analysis in 2005 from McMaster University in Canada showed that melatonin reduced the one-year cancer death by 34 percent across dose range and cancer types without significant side effects. Another meta-analysis of melatonin use in combination with chemotherapy published in the journal of the Danish Medical Association in June 2015 showed that one-year survival of advanced cancers nearly doubled from 28 percent to 52 percent with the use of melatonin.

Mind-body therapy (integrative psychotherapy)

This approach to healing and gaining control over troubling issues works by focusing on a person's capacity for resilience and what resources he or she may have to enable such action. It includes basic principles of traditional psychotherapy and holistic medicine to promote healing on all levels—physical, emotional, mental, and spiritual.

Mind-body therapy aims to create a healthy partnership between one's mind and body. This can happen through various types of counseling services, using tools that may include meditation, visual imagery, or self-expressive writing.

It is common knowledge that our minds can quickly jump to worst-case scenarios, accompanied by anxiety and self-defeating behaviors. Life can become overwhelming; we can waver in our direction and feel as if we've lost our anchor. Any of these emotions or patterns of thought can contribute to illness, compromise relationships, or create a loss of self-esteem.

When a diagnosis of cancer enters someone's life, all of the above comes into play. New patients, feeling more vulnerable than ever before, need all the help they can get. Medicine, nutrition, and supplements play a vital role in the physical healing one needs, but we cannot overlook a patient's mental and emotional health. It is important that we help our patients develop the strength to endure treatment, and that must include the psychological support they need as much as the physical remedies we provide.

Each patient can discover new ways of managing their stress levels while learning how to establish strategies to move forward in a positive manner. It is a process of self-discovery, often under real duress, and doctors can play an instrumental role simply by encouraging their patients to pursue these possibilities.

Cancer treatment creates long-term issues, which may require comprehensive treatment that looks out for the patient's well-being on all levels. Therefore, caring for the mind-body connection is a vital ingredient in creating and maintaining a healthy course of treatment. We encourage our patients to seek out a therapy program that will support them in setting goals, facing fears, developing new daily habits and healthy behaviors, and building the tools they need for healthy communication with their loved ones. Mind-body therapy is used to treat stress and many of the emotions that come along with stress, including a fear of the unknown, which often impair one's ability to create a healthy lifestyle.

Mindfulness-based stress reduction (MBSR)

If you are a person who sometimes longs to shut down your busy brain, this structured program trains you to focus on the present moment and let go of thoughts from the past or worries about the future. MBSR can bring about positive changes, including improved sleep, greater productivity, and both prevention and treatment of chronic illness.

Participating in MBSR is associated with changes in the gray and white matter of the brain, which are involved in learning, memory processes, and emotion regulation. MBSR is used to treat depression, stress, and chronic fatigue syndrome, and can also enhance learning and memory.

Music therapy

Music's powerful effect on the mind transfers easily to the clinical effects on the body. It can influence physical, emotional, cognitive, and social well-being. Listening to music and certain sounds, such as those produced by Tibetan singing bowls, affects various parts of the brain associated with emotion, relaxation, and learning. Music therapy is used to treat depression and high blood pressure, while also enhancing immune function.

Ozone therapy

Ozone, which is triad oxygen ($O3$), supposedly can cause oxidative damage to cancer cells and stunt their growth. It also has been shown to activate immune system cells in increasing the number of WBC and the production of certain immune cytokines such as interferon and IL-2. Ozone is generated in vitro and given intravenously, through rectum or ear canal. It is not recommended for patients with lung cancer due to concerns of lung tissue damage. Although its already very popular with cancer patients seeking alternative cancer care, its value in improving cancer treatment outcomes still needs to be confirmed with further clinical studies.

Qi-gong

This is an ancient, traditional Chinese health care technique. The practice involves a series of postures and exercises, including slow circular movements. It combines relaxation, meditation, and breathing exercises to achieve a tranquil state of mind.

Through study, you learn to manipulate your *Qi*, or life-force energy, to promote healing, prevent disease, and increase longevity. Practitioners of this form believe that this force penetrates and permeates everything in the universe. Qi-gong is used specifically to treat type-2 diabetes and hypertension, as well as to improve bone density. However, its general effects can benefit cancer patients as well.

Reflexology

This form of massage targets reflex points on the feet to cause therapeutic changes in the corresponding organs or body systems. Feet are sensitive to pressure, stretch, and movement. By stimulating their nerve endings with pressure and massage, the body's flow of vital energy can be unblocked. Pressure may also help release pain-altering endorphins in the body. Reflexology is used to treat depression, reduce stress, and post-operative pain, while strengthening the immune function.

Reiki

Originally a 2,500-year-old Buddhist practice, this therapy is based on the belief that the "laying on of hands" can strengthen and normalize certain energy fields within the body and reconnect a person with his or her fundamental life energy. The therapist gently touches your fully clothed body or hovers his or her hands one to two inches above it.

Reiki is a type of biofield therapy and works by encouraging the healing processes of the body and mind, and by restoring and balancing the flow of stagnant energy in the body. The body is thought to regulate the amount of energy it receives and where it goes. Reiki is used to treat depression, stress, and pain relief.

Salt rooms

Salt rooms, also known as halo chambers, are fairly common in Europe and are popping up around the United States, too. They involve soaking in a salt steam bath, or inhaling tiny, breathable salt particles, ground up by machines and dispersed into the air.

Some doctors believe that salt helps respiratory conditions by drawing water into airways, thinning mucus, and improving the function of cilia, the small hairs that help move mucus out of the lungs. Salt rooms are used to treat a range of respiratory ailments, including colds, asthma, allergies, and bronchitis.

Tai chi

Originating as a martial art and sometimes called "moving meditation," this form of exercise is graceful, slow, and low impact. In traditional Chinese medicine, illness is seen as an imbalance between two opposing life forces (yin and yang). Tai chi aims to reestablish that balance to achieve harmony between the body, mind, and outside world. Tai chi is used to treat pain, mood disorders, to control glucose, and to balance problems from Parkinson's disease.

Thalassotherapy

These healing therapies use materials from the sea, such as seaweed body wraps or alluvial mud body scrubs, which contain silt and clay particles. Minerals and trace elements in seawater, absorbed through the skin, are thought to boost the body's blood and lymph circulation to promote the elimination of toxins. Thalassotherapy is used to treat fibromyalgia, dry skin, and to promote and preserve general health.

Western herbal therapy

This therapy uses plants and plant material from seeds, berries, roots, leaves, bark, or flowers to create medicines that help prevent or treat various illnesses. For example, in Germany, the use of herbal therapies, such as St John's Wort for depression, actually exceeds the use of prescribed medications. In fact, many modern medications, like aspirin, are derived from herbs. In fact, the salicylic acid in aspirin comes from tree bark. Western herbal therapy is used to treat insomnia, depression, and circulation problems, as well as to aid in cancer control.

Writing and journaling

Twenty years of research indicates that expressive writing, dealing with one's deepest thoughts and feelings, may contribute to improved physical and emotional health. A 2008 study in *The Oncologist* found that patients who participated in a single twenty-minute writing session improved their outlook on cancer and their overall life quality. [45]

Dr. Daniel Becker, editor of the University of Virginia School of Medicine's *Hospital Drive*, says, "Writing does something to the brain that relieves stress, and unless you get the patient family story right through narrative medicine, you're not going to do an adequate job taking care of them."

Harvard Medical School's *HEALTHbeat* reports, "Writing about thoughts and feelings that arise from a traumatic or stressful life experience—called expressive writing—may help some people cope with the emotional fallout of such events." Writing and journaling is used to treat stress, anxiety, and communication issues.

Yoga

This ancient system of relaxation, exercise, and healing goes back more than five thousand years, with its origins in ancient Indian philosophy. Most Westernized yoga focuses on physical poses, breathing techniques, and meditation, with the goal of achieving relaxation, overall health, and improved fitness.

Long, deep breathing encourages the actions of the parasympathetic nervous system, the system that lowers blood pressure and slows our breathing, allowing for relaxation and healing to take place. Yoga also tones and strengthens our entire body, especially the core, which is especially helpful for people who may not favor going to a gym. Yoga is used to treat stress, insomnia, mood swings, and chronic pain.

LESSONS TO LEARN FROM TREATING THE IMMUNE SYSTEM WITH INTEGRATIVE THERAPY

Consider what happens when a patient with advanced cancer goes into remission. It's very likely that cancer cells remain in his or her body, and with modern technology you can sometimes find actual traces of cancer markers even when it seems that the treatment has eradicated the disease. MTD chemotherapy would be too toxic to continue treating the cancer at this stage. Without integrative therapies, all a patient can do is to wait for outright recurrences or progression before restarting treatment. This is exactly what Ted, a patient with incompletely resected pancreatic cancer with rapid rising tumor marker readings but no clearly detectable cancer, was told to do by a local pancreatic cancer specialist.

Ted was diagnosed with pancreatic tail adenocarcinoma about six years ago. Pancreatic cancer from this location is notoriously known to be found at a late stage since there are no major early warning symptoms. Ted underwent surgical resection but apparently, the surgeon failed to remove it completely (positive surgical margin), and Ted's cancer markers started to go up very rapidly within weeks after surgery. He was having some small dots of lesions in his liver, which we treated with low-dose chemotherapy. Initially, it all went away, but from time to time, every three to six months, the cancer marker would start to shoot up very rapidly, indicating the cancer was starting to come back. I would then treat him with almost the same regimen as I had several times before, and his numbers would go back down. We kept doing scans, and every time his cancer marker went up, we couldn't find his cancer or any other reason why the markers kept going up.

That was the case until the technology of the liquid biopsy was developed. The next time his cancer marker went up quickly, we analyzed his blood for specific mutations that only cancer cells carry. I wasn't surprised to find that lots of tumor DNAs were in his blood correlating with the cancer activity detected by the tumor marker.

If we had not treated it right then, it would have become a full-blown case, and the chance for him to survive beyond five years would have been almost zero after the unsuccessful surgery. With MLDC, Ted was able to tolerate repeated prolonged chemotherapy sessions without enduring major side effects. Ted's integrative therapy plan included low-dose interferon, regular high-dose intravenous vitamin C, multiple immune-supporting supplements, medical cannabis, acupuncture, diet, and exercise. Today, Ted continues to live a vibrant life, including work as a spiritual psychologist, advocating for the welfare of local homeless people, and avid jogging on a daily basis.

That brings us to the matter of the immune system. Why is it, after all these treatments over the last several years, that Ted's cancer has come back less and less? Normally, an oncologist believes that a cancer will come back stronger and stronger with subsequent recurrences occurring over shorter and shorter intervals. But in Ted's case, we have reversed the pattern. The cancer keeps coming back less and less frequently, and eventually seems as though it has been eliminated. I have seen this happen in other patients, too. Although this has not invalidated the theory that one with advanced cancer can never be cured, it is starting to push the boundaries of this clinical dogma.

I think the MLDC (in the form of combination chemotherapy when cancer was active and maintenance oral cyclophosphamide when in remission) in combination with immune-supportive integrative therapies had gradually shifted the balance between the immune system and the cancer, leading to the eventual retake of cancer control inside the patient's body. Importantly, the chemotherapy itself did not generate drug resistance during treatment, unlike what usually occurs during a traditional course of MTD chemotherapy. Ted's story shows again the wisdom of taking care of the immune system.

Terry is a vibrant fifty-two-year-old woman with two young daughters and a very supportive husband. She was originally diagnosed with stage IIb ER/PR positive and HER-2/Neu positive breast cancer in early 2001. She underwent a lumpectomy followed by conventional adjuvant chemotherapy and radiation at a large local hospital. She developed recurrent metastatic breast cancer to multiple bony areas while taking tamoxifen in 2005 and was treated with low-dose chemotherapy in conjunction with Herceptin and ovarian ablation. Seeing the cancer come back so quickly after going through all the heavy treatments, Terry intuitively knew she needed to do something more than just drug therapy.

After extensive research of her own she inquired about intravenous vitamin C as an adjunctive therapy but was told with no equivocal tones that this was not something that the large medical center would offer. Determined, Terry switched her care to see me at Seattle Cancer Treatment and Wellness Center, where intravenous vitamin C was embraced as a complementary therapy for cancer. Under the guidance of the center's naturopathic doctor, she received weekly high-dose intravenous vitamin C infusions while continuing the Herceptin and adding a slew of supplements to support her immune system and decrease inflammation. She also started a ketogenic diet that she follows at least 80 percent of the time.

She joined several supportive groups to share her experience and fear with other patients in similar situations. Over the next twelve years, Terry's cancer stayed in her bones and remained mostly stable. After a recent surgery to remove a relatively large skull lesion, repeated PET-CT scans appeared to show less and less cancerous activity in her bones and nowhere else. She has traveled extensively over the years and continues to live a vibrant life of family and volunteering to help others in need.

Terry's cancer returned less than four years after initial diagnosis of early stage breast cancer treated with conventional surgery, radiation, and high-dose chemotherapy but has remained stable with bone-involving stage 4 disease over the last twelve years without significant disease progression on an integrative treatment plan as discussed above. Her case reemphasizes the notion that by supporting a patient's immune system while suppressing cancer growth with integrative therapies, we can turn a potentially aggressive cancer into a chronic disease that we can manage on an ongoing basis.

The Goal of Integrative Cancer Treatments

We have seen in this chapter how we aim to improve our patients' sense of well-being and quality of life after a cancer diagnosis by reducing stress, improving their nutritional status and immune system function, as well as boosting their tolerance levels for conventional treatments. By integrating any and all of these therapies, we are increasing our patients' chances of finding success with their treatment regimens, both to curtail the cancer and to set up a lifelong path for better health.

INTEGRATIVE MEDICINE RESOURCES

We suggest the following resources for additional follow-up:

> Society of Integrative Oncology
> Oncology Association of Naturopathic Physicians (ONCANP)
> Bastyr University

We also encourage you to seek out integrative oncologists, MDs trained in integrative medicine, and naturopathic physicians to be on your team of doctors for the best cancer treatment outcomes.

5

INTEGRATIVE TREATMENT PLANS IN ACTION

Case Histories and Statistics

When I was a medical school resident at the University of Nebraska Medical Center, I was contemplating doing a fellowship in medical oncology later and asked my mentor, Dr. James Armitage, what he thought about the job market for a medical oncologist. He jokingly replied that while there are a lot of oncologists, there are not enough good oncologists. His comments, and his example as a compassionate leading cancer physician, inspired me to be better at what I do and to pursue being the best. This desire accompanied me when I became the research director at Seattle Cancer Treatment and Wellness Center, the former northwestern affiliate of Cancer Treatment Centers of America.

Early on during the nearly twelve years I worked there, I began to learn about low-dose chemotherapy, especially from Dr. Ben Chue, who was there a few years before me and was starting to use more and more of the method. Although my training focused solely on MTD (maximum tolerated dosing) chemotherapy during my fellowship, I was very intrigued by some of the methods he started to use and the surprisingly good results he got on some very difficult-to-treat patients. In 2006, we coauthored a report to the year's American Society of Clinical Oncology (ASCO) meeting on four very advanced pancreatic cancer patients, three of whom had failed at least one line of previous chemotherapy and were dangerously jaundiced. The low-dose combination chemotherapy protocol that Dr. Chue and I reported for these pancreatic cancer patients was remarkably effective; their CA19.9 and bilirubin levels fell to near normal ranges in a matter of weeks. Although a subsequent effort to conduct a formal clinical trial did not come to fruition due to lack of research funding, this protocol is still being used in our clinic for the benefit of many subsequent patients.

Initially, a metronomically modified conventional regime was used for those patients who had failed or couldn't tolerate an MTD regimen. These protocols were commonly acceptable alternative regimens to the MTD protocol (e.g., weekly Taxol and carboplatin versus Taxol and carboplatin once every three weeks), but were often reserved for weak or elderly patients deemed too weak to tolerate intensive chemotherapy. But as we gave these less intensive treatments to our patients more consistently, we started to see better and better outcomes. Over the years, it became almost an exception *not* to see a favorable response in patients with all the common types of cancer we treated. Many of them had already failed one or more lines of treatment outside of our center. Still, I found that patients who came to us first had the best outcomes, often achieving long remissions. As the gap between the treatment results from metronomic protocols and conventional protocols became larger and larger, I could not in all conscience go back to an MTD-based practice.

Our use of MLDC (metronomic low-dose chemotherapy) was also driven by the type of patients who came to the Cancer Treatment Centers of America (CTCA) for a different cancer care experience. These patients were usually very well educated and holistically oriented people, who had generally lived a healthy lifestyles and had a natural concern about any kind of drugs. We had many patients coming to us determined to forgo *any* chemotherapy. Some of them had already experienced horrible side effects from conventional chemotherapy received at a cancer center that, in the end, could no longer help them. So these patients were making appointments at CTCA, hoping we could offer something different. Some of them were intent on doing nothing but natural medicine. But we knew in most cases natural medicine alone would not be enough.

We also had people brought in by family members seeking a last resort, hoping that some last-ditch effort would save their loved ones. We tried to help, but the conventional options are limited when a patient is already weakened and malnourished from both cancer and previous treatments, when their blood count is down to levels that do not permit any further chemotherapy, or when they are too depressed to have the will to fight. You can only overcome so much damage. The immune system can be built back up, but it's a slow, gradual process. If the cancer has already been raging in the body for a long time in the absence of any effective treatments and complementary supportive therapies, it's a huge challenge. Still, as we changed the direction of treatments for these patients, some of them started to improve. Sometimes, even when these improvements were mild and transient, they improved the patient's quality of life and provided great comforts to the family. Other times, these improvements continued to get bigger until, like the pancreatic cancer patients described above, they miraculously achieved a lasting remission.

At the time, our center had more naturopaths than oncologists, and it was in that environment with increasing experiences that I started to see that metronomic low-dose chemotherapy was not only reasonable; it represented a better way than MTD chemotherapy to control cancer, especially when combined with complementary naturopathic medicine.

DISCOVERING A BETTER MODEL

Metronomic low-dose chemotherapy has a strong scientific base from decades of research.[1] Even though it has been eclipsed by the MTD approach in the general oncology community, it is a viable option for many patients. The drugs used are all FDA approved for particular cancer types. Clinical data has accumulated showing that when these drugs are administered in low doses on a regular basis, the outcomes are often better than typical MTD chemotherapy using the very same drugs.[2] As expected, the lower dose is also associated with significantly reduced side effects,[3] which improves the overall quality of life of patients and facilitates their effort to become stronger both physically and mentally to rise to the monumental challenge of defeating cancer.

When combined with support from naturopathic medicine, the results of MLDC are often remarkable. On the surface you can see patients who are getting better in many ways, mind and body. Inside, it is their own innate fighting power that is getting stronger with the help of a gentle treatment and other measures designed specifically to support the immune system. This is one situation where theories support practice, and practice corroborates theory.

In late 2002, I began treating Ellen, who was seventy-five years old at the time, quite frail, and suffering from stage 4 lung cancer that had spread to her lungs, the lymphatic system in her chest, and her adrenal gland. Her first oncologist had told her that she probably had nine months to live. Her husband was also very ill, so she was stressed out, and obviously would have done poorly on any regimen of high-dose chemotherapy. I took a leap of faith with Ellen because I had recently seen some data on the effects of low doses of chemotherapy administered on a weekly basis. So I treated her with weekly low-dose chemotherapy, and we took care of her body by having her see the naturopath to support her with diet, nutrition, and certain supplements.

Ellen responded well and, after several weeks, she showed real signs of improvement. Her nasty cough was much better, and the cancer, which had originally appeared as a sprinkling of black dots on PET-CT scans, was getting lighter and lighter, and some of the dots started to disappear. At the time, the conventional wisdom was that you could only treat a patient with four to six cycles of high-dose chemotherapy before the benefits ended. Any more cycles hurt more than helped because of the accumulation of side effects.

But it was different with Ellen. She just kept getting better and better, with mild and manageable side effects. She was able to continue her low-dose treatment for a whole nine months. The cancer did not go away completely, but scans at three-month intervals showed steady improvement. Finally, just before we reached the twelve-month mark, all traces of the cancer completely disappeared. Between two years and five years after we began treating her, the cancer came back but on a smaller scale. Each time she was given the same treatment she received when she first came to us, and both times she went back into remission. After she achieved remission for the second recurrence, she was placed on the maintenance drug Tarceva, which had just become available. She remained in remission for another five years before another spot of cancer came back in her lung. A biopsy showed that it was the same poorly differentiated lung adenocarcinoma. But now, with a new understanding of the molecular biology of lung cancer, we determined that cancer came in two genetic forms, one of which made the cancer resistant to the drug Tarceva. Ellen had that variant. She was then treated with a new targeted drug called Tagrisso, which was effective for the new mutation, but unfortunately this drug gave her more side effects than chemotherapy. Without consistent treatment, her cancer progressed, eventually causing a severe shortness of breath from the accumulation of malignant fluids in her lungs. At age eighty-eight, nearly fifteen years after the initial diagnosis of stage 4 lung cancer, Ellen asked to restart her low-dose chemotherapy for the fourth time. As of this writing, Ellen's stage 4 lung cancer had gone into a fourth complete remission as confirmed by PET-CT scans, and again Ellen has tolerated the treatment mostly well.

Ellen's success in treating her lung cancer shows that MLDC can be given over a much longer period of time than MTD chemotherapy to induce remission gradually and without debilitating side effects. It also shows that repeated cycles of MLDC do not induce drug resistance like MTD chemotherapy in cancer cells, a phenomenon that was also seen in Ted Jenkins, whose case history was discussed in chapter 3.

Over the years, Ellen's success provided guidance for me as I worked with numerous other patients with similar stage 4 lung cancers. Although Ellen's good long-term outcome is exceptional, I continue to have consistent success in treating patients like Ellen—nearly 100 percent for a while, until one very ill patient came in to break the streak. Still, I estimate that over 90 percent of my advanced lung cancer patients have benefited from the treatments. Their median survival tripled the national average, reaching three years in 2008, when I reported my results at the International Lung Cancer Congress held in Maui, Hawaii.[4] This was at a time before any of the immunotherapy drugs currently available had been developed.

Ellen's successful treatment, and successes with a mounting number of patients with similar conditions, fueled a growing confidence in a metronomic approach to chemotherapy. *Less is more.* If treatment is gentle, steady, and consistent, it can bring cancer under control without causing undue harm. This is how MLDC works, and how it works in concert with the immune system.

Cancer can erupt again and again, somewhat like a forest fire. Some trees truly burn out while others smolder silently, bursting back into flame when conditions permit. But as long as we have a good control and monitoring system, we can manage these flare-ups and prevent them from growing into a major conflagration.

ON THE RIGHT TRACK TO LONG-TERM CANCER
CONTROL: INDIVIDUAL CASE HISTORIES

Over the years I have been amazed by the striking responses and continuous improvement of cancer control in some of my patients with advanced cancers.

Olga was an otherwise healthy twenty-one-year-old woman when she was diagnosed with aggressive lymphoma of the chest (mediastinal diffuse large B-cell lymphoma) seven years ago. She was treated at a large cancer center with standard R-CHOP regimen. She only had a partial response and was monitored. Less than two years later, her cancer progressed with repeated growth in her chest that spread to her spine. She was then treated at the same center with a more aggressive high-dose salvage chemotherapy regimen called EPOCH. After two cycles, she experienced increasing pain to her chest and lower back. A repeat PET-CT scan showed her cancer had gotten worse with the treatment. She was told she might need radiation and surgery to prevent further complications from the advancing cancer, but the risk of side effects from these procedures was equally high. At that time Olga found us and decided to give our integrative therapy a try. We immediately started her on a low-dose biochemotherapy regimen using gemcitabine, cisplatin, dexamethasone and rituximab (Rituxan), along with high-dose intravenous vitamin C. Her pain improved dramatically after just one to two treatments. After three months, a repeat PET-CT scan showed that her lymphoma that never responded to the high-dose chemotherapy was almost completely gone. She continued with a maintenance of high-dose vitamin C infusion therapy. Five years later, repeated scans showed Olga has remained in complete remission. She was pregnant twice during this time and had two healthy babies, whom she still found good energy to take care of. Olga's case exemplifies what integrative treatment combining MLDC and complementary therapies can do where conventional medicine has failed.

Recently, another young woman came to me with the same diagnosis. She also had failed two previous lines of conventional high-dose chemotherapy with progressive symptoms. After going through the same treatment that Olga did for six weeks, her chest pain resolved, and she could sleep better on her back. A repeat CT scan showed that her large chest lymphoma mass had already decreased by more than half and some smaller lymph nodes had disappeared. In writing these cases, I can't help wondering how many patients like Olga are out there, patients who didn't know about us and have died unnecessarily? I have presented our successful lymphoma treatment experiences to Society of Integrative Oncology (SIO). I am writing this book, and I will keep writing reports. I am hopeful that the world will start to take notice soon.

Bruce is a long-term pancreatic cancer patient of mine. In May of 2010, after months of unsuccessful attempts to get a diagnosis for severe stomach and back pain and digestive problems, he discovered that he had inoperable stage 3 pancreatic cancer. Physicians at both the Swedish Hospital in Seattle and the Mayo Clinic in Scottsdale, Arizona, advised him to get his affairs in order, because he "was on a short path." A physician at the Swedish Hospital told him he had six to eight months with treatment, and considerably less without.

Refusing to give up so easily, he sought a second opinion from CTCA, where I worked at the time. When I first saw him, he was sixty-two years old and generally in good health except for his cancer. During our first meetings, I discovered that his lifestyle already included many of the elements we recommend: his diet was heavy in fruits, vegetables, and fish; he regularly took immune supporting supplements (e.g., curcumin, melatonin, mushroom extracts, etc.), and he exercised and meditated regularly. Because there was no evidence that the cancer had spread to distant areas at the time, his initial treatment was a combination of low-dose weekly gemcitabine and radiation to the pancreatic tumor.

After five months of this regimen, his cancer markers had declined significantly, but he was not yet in remission. I then put him on a weekly MLDC program of oxaliplatin and 5-FU. Unfortunately, after only two cycles of this program, Bruce suffered a cardiac event, very similar to a heart attack, called "stress cardiomyopathy" or "Takotsubo cardiomyopathy" because the left ventricle comes to look like a wide, traditional Japanese octopus trap. This type of non-ischemic cardiomyopathy is triggered by overwhelming emotional stress, such as the death of a loved one, a break-up, or constant anxiety. In Bruce's case, the source of the stress was the diagnosis of pancreatic cancer (then considered a death sentence), the recent loss of a job, and perhaps a sensitivity to 5-FU. Bruce suffered his cardiac event in January of 2011, recovered, and attempted to resume treatment in late February of 2011. However, my colleagues and I did not think it was prudent to resume treatment so soon after a near-fatal event, so we placed him on a monitoring program. After a series of CT scans showed a slight decrease in size of the pancreatic tumor, and the CA19.9 cancer marker fell to level of nondetectability, Bruce was declared in remission. This near total remission lasted for five years, during which time Bruce and his wife resumed the outdoor activities and travel they had enjoyed before. The only concessions he made to cancer during this time were periodic CT scans and blood tests for the CA19.9 cancer marker. This resumption of an active life occurred despite a mild stroke he suffered in the fall of 2012. Bruce recovered quickly from this setback, with no permanent effects except a mild speech impediment usually undetectable to others.

However, in April of 2016, a small mass in his left lung that had long been visible in CT scans suddenly increased in size at the same time that the CA19.9 cancer marker shot up. A biopsy confirmed that the mass was metastatic pancreatic cancer. I placed him on a weekly MLDC regimen of vitamin C, Gemzar, and Abraxane, a drug in the Taxol family. Bruce's cancer markers fell steadily and in July of 2016, he once again achieved partial remission. However, unlike most of my patients, Bruce developed relatively severe neuropathy in response to the Abraxane. These symptoms decreased somewhat during the remission, during which time he followed a maintenance program of low-dose interferon injections, oral cyclophosphamide, and a variety of supplements intended to bolster his immune system (curcumin, mushroom extracts, the Ayurvedic herb mixture called triphala, etc.).

In March of 2017, his cancer markers once more shot up, and I placed him on an MLDC regimen of intravenous vitamin C, Gemzar, and cisplatin (Abraxane was dropped because of his sensitivity to that drug). At the time of this writing, Bruce's cancer markers are still elevated, but they appear to have leveled off. His treatment is complicated somewhat by periodic depressions in white blood cells or platelets, conditions which cause him to skip infusions. Nevertheless there is every reason to hope he will once again achieve remission, as he has done twice before. Meanwhile, Bruce is living a fairly active life limited only by the persistent neuropathy brought about by Abraxane.

Bruce's case is remarkable because it shows that an integrative cancer control program can succeed in providing long-lasting control of a very serious cancer even in the face of multiple, non-cancer-related diseases and the development of significant side effects.

Amphone is another patient I have seen for over ten years. When I first saw her, she had large lymph nodes blossoming in her groin and abdomen from follicular lymphoma associated with generalized weakness, night sweats, and indigestion. She was treated with metronomic R-CHOP and had near complete response. However, Amphone endured major recurrences every two to three years. Each time I was able to put her back into remission by administering a gentle form of weekly chemo combined with immunotherapy Rituxan and a steady regimen of weekly vitamin C infusions and multiple supplements she received from our naturopath. She also seeks out other sources of supportive care, including acupuncture, yoga, and meditation. This combined effort of treatment and support worked well for her, and she lived actively through the years, including seeing two kids through college, gardening, and extensive overseas traveling.

On the fifteenth anniversary of being diagnosed with an incurable cancer, one expected to become steadily more aggressive, Amphone actually achieved the best state of remission yet: all her lymphoma-involved lymph nodes normalized completely on her most recent scan. This result goes completely against expectations for follicular lymphoma, and there is no explanation for it except that her immune system finally overcame the cancer with the help of our treatments and support.

This is not an isolated case by any means. In the patient case report of over one hundred subjects with different lymphomas I presented to the SIO conference (Society for Integrative Oncology) in 2014, most had achieved similarly good outcomes.

Richard is a soft-spoken sixty-eight-year-old man with colon cancer diagnosed nearly thirteen years ago. When I first saw him, he had rectal bleeding and pain. After a colonoscopy, he was diagnosed with locally invasive rectal cancer. He underwent initial treatment with chemoradiation and was then advised to have surgery. However, because he was told the location of his cancer would force him to wear a colostomy bag for the rest of his life after surgery, he hesitated and sought a second opinion, while receiving additional radiation treatment with gamma knife.

Within a year, his cancer progressed and he started bleeding again. At that time he came to see me, still opposed to having any surgery that would entail a colostomy. Since his risk of metastases was very high at that time due to the delay in undergoing surgery, I started him on systemic chemotherapy using metronomic weekly oxaliplatin and 5-FU. He responded very well to this treatment: his bleeding stopped, and the repeat colonoscopy four months later showed his cancer was in remission.

He remained in remission for the next five years with no signs of either local or distant recurrence, until his rectal pain started again. Work-up showed he had a local recurrence of the cancer. At this time he decided to have surgery done, but the cancer was found to have metastasized into his abdomen causing a small bowel obstruction. He was then treated with the same metronomic chemotherapy for three months. He then finally consented to the surgery to remove the tumor and to perform a colostomy. Miraculously, no intra-abdominal disease was found at that time.

He has remained on a maintenance therapy for the last five years consisting of metronomic antiangiogenic therapy with low-dose oral Xeloda and Avastin, and he has never had another recurrence. Thirteen years later, he is finally healthy and well. He told me that since he was diagnosed with cancer, he was told six times that he was terminal and he should get his affairs in order. If he had listened to any one of those advisors, he would not be alive today.

In addition to metronomic chemotherapy, he had followed naturopathic recommendations with alternating batteries of supplements, daily doses of flaxseed oil, vitamin D3, and melatonin. He also alternates different supplements including spirulina, mushroom extracts, turmeric, and MSM to explore the optimal benefits in boosting his immune system and cutting down on inflammation.

This case illustrates that the combination of metronomic chemotherapy and complementary naturopathic medicine can put cancer into long-lasting remission, and turn a potentially life-threatening disease into a chronic disease that can be monitored and managed.

Phoumy is a fifty-two-year-old physician's assistant who worked with a well-known hematologist in a major medical center. In April of 2010 he came down with an illness that made him extremely tired, and he also developed enlarged lymph nodes in his neck. A subsequent workup by his hematologist showed that he had developed a very complicated case of lymphoma including a stage 1 diffuse large B cell lymphoma and a stage 4 T-cell lymphoma that infiltrated his bone marrow and the surface of the spinal cord. He was treated with conventional regimen of R-CHOP (rituximab, cyclophosphamide, doxorubicin, vincristine, and prednisone) for six cycles. Post-treatment evaluation showed that his diffuse large B-cell lymphoma in the lymph nodes appeared to have gone into remission, but he had significant residual T-cell lymphoma in his bone marrow. In light of the fact his T-cell disease was slow-growing at that time, he was placed on watch for monitoring without further treatment.

After six years of remission, in October 2016, Phoumy had major progression of the T-cell lymphoma with a dangerously elevated calcium level in his blood with multiple swollen lymph nodes in his abdomen and a swollen spleen. He was hospitalized and treated with an aggressive high-dose chemotherapy regimen called EPOCH that lasts for five days each time and repeats every three weeks. After two rounds of treatment, he became severely debilitated with diffuse muscle aches, stiffness, and extreme difficulty walking. Repeat PET scan showed that his cancer had merely remained stable.

At that time, his treatment was switched to another high-dose protocol combining four different chemotherapy drugs. The plan was to treat him with this regimen for a few cycles, then to do a bone marrow transplantation. Due to the side effects Phoumy had already experienced, he decided to discontinue this treatment.

Phoumy came to see me in January 2017 with a repeat PET scan showing that his cancer had already progressed from when he was first diagnosed with recurrent disease in October 2016. He was started on a weekly metronomic low-dose chemotherapy with gemcitabine and cisplatin along with high-dose intravenous vitamin C infusion and a battery of supplements including reishi mushrooms and vitamin D3. Phoumy quickly stabilized, the side effects of his previous chemotherapy disappeared, and he started to feel like his old self again. Three months after the treatment, a repeat CT scan showed that all the severely enlarged lymph nodes in various parts of his body, including the abdomen and retroperitoneal space, had nearly all resolved. He continued on his high-dose intravenous vitamin C infusions and felt so well that he decided to take a trip to Hawaii and then to Thailand to visit temples there for meditation and massage therapy. He came back refreshed, and a repeat PET scan in August of 2017 showed his cancer remained in complete remission. He resumed his vitamin C infusions and continued with other supplements to support his immune system. I last saw him in mid-October, and he felt so well that he was ready to go back to work as a physician's assistant, this time with the state department of health.

Phoumy told me that he has continued to see his previous doctor and has retained a good relationship with him. Letters from the doctor indicated that he was very pleased but a bit puzzled with the progress Phoumy has made with the "alternative care" that he has received. Nonetheless, he now completely supports the direction Phoumy has taken and encourages him to continue to see me.

This case illustrates that in the face of a very aggressive form of lymphoma where even more aggressive high-dose chemotherapy had failed, low-dose metronomic chemotherapy in combination with intravenous vitamin C did wonders, inducing complete response associated with a much better quality of life. Maintenance therapy, with high-dose intravenous vitamin C and natural supplements that boost the immune system, has kept Phoumy in remission without continuous treatment.

Randy is a long-term survivor of stage 4 gastroesophageal cancer with metastases to the liver and lymph nodes. He is also an energetic and outspoken man, with three small children, a strong religious faith, a commissioner with a south Seattle port authority, a member of the local county planning commission, a Habitat for Humanity volunteer, and a real estate broker.

When his cancer was first diagnosed, the tumor in his lower esophagus was huge, and in CT scans Randy says it "looked like a cauliflower in my throat." Randy's throat was almost closed off by the tumor and swallowing was very difficult and very painful. Biopsy confirmed it was a cancer called poorly differentiated gastroesophageal junction adenocarcinoma. A PET-CT scan showed that cancer had already spread to the liver. Diagnosed in April of 2011 at the age of forty-eight, his first doctor told Randy he would likely be dead by June. Nevertheless this oncologist suggested treating the tumor with radiation to see if it could relieve the obstruction. But the oncologist also pointed out that any relief from radiation to this large tumor would likely be very temporary, and if radiation caused sores on the surface of his esophagus, his swallowing difficulty might even get worse. Moreover, radiation treatment was not going to help with his metastatic liver tumor, which would likely spread further. Advised to get a second opinion, Randy contacted me.

After meeting me, Randy was very impressed with the additional options that he had not heard before, options that also made a lot of sense for him. He decided to forgo the radiation treatment for a while and gave our integrative treatment plan a try. He agreed to have a temporary feeding tube placed if necessary. Randy said he was ready to do whatever was necessary and to do it quickly—which was clearly necessary for someone in Randy's desperate condition when I first saw him.

I decided to treat him with a multidrug metronomic chemotherapy protocol that we had already used with great success in the treatment of various gastrointestinal malignancies. He also received intravenous glutathione, an antioxidant that has also been shown to prevent peripheral nerve damage from certain chemotherapy agents.

After just one treatment, his swallowing pain was a little better. He continued to improve every week with the treatment, and by the end of three months his swallowing had nearly all normalized. A repeat PET-CT scan showed very minimal residual cancer activity at his primary tumor site but the metastatic lesions had completely disappeared. After continuing treatment for another six weeks he underwent another EGD (esophagogastroduodenoscopy, examination of esophagus, stomach, and small intestine by scoped camera). To the surprise of the gastroenterologist, no signs of tumor could be found at the esophageal site this time. He took a biopsy at the tumor site and the microscopic examination of the tissue also showed no cancer. His cancer had gone into a complete remission. Diagnosed with terminal cancer in April and in complete remission by early November!

We decided to stop the chemotherapy at that time and started him on a newly approved monoclonal antibody therapy called Herceptin (trastuzumab). This antibody binds to the overproduced HER-2 protein on the surface of cancer cells and delivers an inhibitory signal to them. Herceptin is also an immunotherapy that can induce an immune attack on cancer cells called antibody-dependent cytotoxicity.

Randy has shown no sign of cancer since he went on the maintenance treatment. Subsequent biopsies of the lower esophagus were all negative for any residual or recurrent cancer, and so were the repeated imaging scans. His health recovered quickly after finishing the chemotherapy. Indeed, his health never really deteriorated all that much even *during* therapy: Randy maintained his busy life, including a very contentious wrangle over a sewer project on the Port Commission, throughout the first eight months of his treatment. Six years after his diagnosis of stage 4 gastroesophageal cancer, Randy has remained healthy and cancer free.

This is a remarkable and inspiring story of cancer recovery helped by metronomic low-dose chemotherapy and immunotherapy. It underscores the power of this integrative approach that can put even advanced cancer into durable, long-lasting remission along with gains of quality of life that may even be better than before the cancer diagnosis.

Susan is a mother, a grandmother, and a lifetime horse person with a handsome black stallion show horse that she is proud to show around the country from time to time. She says she is not a worrier and approaches life very proactively. She is a believer in the interactive benefit of diet (she diligently avoids sugar since her diagnosis), exercise, and selected supplements. When she found a mass on her right breast almost twelve years ago, she quickly went through breast examinations with a mammogram, and then an ultrasound-guided biopsy, which soon returned an unequivocal diagnosis of breast cancer estrogen and progesterone receptors positive and HER-2 receptor positive.

HER-2 positive cancer is a more aggressive form of breast cancer due to the overexpression of HER-2 protein on the cancer cell's surface that autonomously drive the cancer growth. A CT scan for staging showed that the cancer had spread to her liver with a 2-cm lesion. Under the recommendation of a naturopathic physician, Susan came to see me for further evaluation and treatment. Considering that her cancer likely had already spread to her liver, I advised her to start on systemic chemotherapy first. She agreed and started on a weekly metronomic chemotherapy protocol alone with Herceptin. Three months later, a repeat breast MRI and an abdominal CT scan showed that all her cancers were gone and she had attained a complete remission. She decided to forgo surgery on her breast at that time because clinical studies I reviewed with her showed no improvement in survival in patients with stage 4 breast cancer. She continued her treatment with Herceptin and added an antiestrogen medication.

Her cancer remained in remission for the next six years, when suddenly her blood cancer marker started to climb rapidly. A CT scan showed that numerous cancerous lesions in her liver as well as signs of metastatic cancer in her lymph nodes and bones. A biopsy of the liver lesion was positive for metastatic breast cancer but, unlike the first, it was HER-2 negative. The cancer likely had mutated or lost its HER-2 expression.

She was restarted on the same weekly metronomic chemotherapy regimen. Remarkably, she again attained complete remission four months later. During this time, and through the entire period of the second round of chemotherapy, Susan felt a mysterious calm, even joyfulness. She says she intuitively "knew" she would be okay, and she was looking forward to seeing what God had in store for her.

After she entered remission, she was placed on a targeted therapy drug called Afinitor (everolimus) combined with a different antiestrogen drug. Although she did not tolerate Afinitor very well, and I had to cut back her dose by half, her breast cancer has not returned. Now, nearly twelve years after her first diagnosis of stage 4 cancer—and many horse shows—she remains healthy and optimistic.

Susan's story exemplifies the great success we had in managing breast cancer. For an overview of the success we have had treating breast cancer, please read the statistical summary in our reports to SIO in 2013 documenting the outcomes my patients have attained with various stages of and types of breast cancer. All of these patients were treated with metronomic low-dose chemotherapy embedded in an integrative treatment.

The treatment I gave my long-term patients are not drastically different from conventional protocols in that I usually use the same FDA approved drugs and combinations but just give them in more sensible doses and more consistent frequencies. These simple changes in combination with complementary supportive therapies seem all that it takes to make big differences in my patients, many with very difficult cancers that don't bear good outcomes with conventional treatments at all.

The problems we are facing today are increasingly decreased physician autonomy in making treatment decisions, which instead are being increasingly controlled by rigid guidelines based on outdated MTD principle and insurance payment polices, mostly aimed at controlling cost. For myself, I often find it difficult to give my patients MTD chemotherapy out of good conscience, but more often than I'd like, a compromise must be made to provide any patient treatment at all. For the sake of our patients, for whom we care about, urgent action is needed. We must reexamine our chemotherapy approach and embrace the patient as a whole person, body and spirit, to help them survive and thrive.

Scientific studies have shown that MTD chemotherapy is usually associated with prolonged suppression of patients' native immune function, including NK cells and CD8 T-cell activities. [5] The reason my patients' cancers continue to recede and eventually disappear is that the integrated treatment has not only repeatedly beaten back the cancer, it has also built up their antitumor immune response. Every time the cancer is treated, antigens are released that can be recognized by the immune system. Because metronomic low-dose chemotherapy modifies the immune system to favor the antitumor response, a combination of MLDC and other holistic ways of boosting the immune system progressively strengthens the immune system until the cancer is totally controlled.

The few patients who came to me after heavy and prolonged MTD chemotherapy without any complementary therapies sometimes couldn't handle more treatment of any kind. Cancer had almost completely overpowered their chemo-blasted immune systems. No external treatment can help for very long. This sad status quo cannot be changed by introducing more and more pharmaceutical drugs aiming at smaller and smaller targets. Fundamental changes to our thinking and approach to basic cancer care need to happen quickly to save more lives.

Beyond the scientific analysis, MLDC is just common sense. We must reach a median: poison the body a little bit to get rid of the cancer but not enough to damage our own inner fighting power, which we all believe in now. MLDC and integrative therapies are perfect solutions to this equation. We will give our patients a fighting chance from the beginning by not administering too high a dose of chemotherapy. Instead, we bolster the immune system and other organs with a synergistic integrative treatment plan. With one hand, we're hitting the cancer with metronomic low-dose chemotherapy, which beats it back steadily and consistently, while with the other hand we support and strengthen the patient with a wide array of supplemental treatments.

ON THE RIGHT TRACK TO LONG-TERM CANCER CONTROL: STATISTICS

Having looked in detail at the results individual patients have received with integrative MLDC, it is instructive to evaluate this therapy from a statistical perspective, looking at the response of groups of patients suffering from the same or related cancers, receiving various forms of integrative MLDC. For this purpose, we will look at the responses of seventy-five women with early stages of breast cancer, and thirty-seven with stage 4 disease. We will also look at the results of treating twenty-four patients suffering various forms of non-Hodgkin's lymphoma with MLDC and high-dose intravenous vitamin C.

BREAST CANCER STATISTICS

Breast cancer treatment still faces significant challenges from both treatment failure and treatment-related side effects. According to national statistics, patients diagnosed with stage 1 and 2 breast cancer who receive conventional treatments have about a 20 percent risk of recurrence and 80 to 90 percent survival after five years. Patients with stage 3 breast cancer have worse prognosis, with a median five-year survival rate between 40 and 66 percent. Patients with stage 4 breast cancer have the worst prognosis, with a median survival time of less than two years, and an estimated five-year survival rate of about 15 percent.[6]

I have personally treated and followed 112 breast cancer patients who received integrated therapies including conventional treatments with surgery, chemotherapy, radiation, and antiestrogen therapy, and complementary therapies including naturopathic medicine and acupuncture. For chemotherapy treatment, patients typically receive MLDC to reduce the treatment toxicity and to improve dose density. The naturopathic treatments patients receive are designed to boost antitumor immune response and to suppress inflammation and consist of a core group of supplements modified as necessary to suit individual patients.

Patients in the analysis were treated from 2005 through 2012. All of these patients received majority of their treatments in our clinic under my care and the care of a group of naturopathic physicians. A total of forty-eight patients with stage 1 and 2 breast cancers were followed for a median of five years. Only two of these patients (4.7 percent) developed distant recurrences, and none of the patients have died from their disease. Of twenty-seven patients with stage 3 breast cancer that have been followed for a median of 3.5 years, three (11 percent) developed distant recurrences and only one (3.7 percent) died of the disease. Of the thirty-seven patients with stage 4 breast cancer, the estimated five-year survival rate is 53 percent, and median survival time is 5.8 years.

The data indicates that the integrated treatment model discussed above can lead to excellent clinical outcomes in breast cancer patients. The data in Figure 5.1 and in Tables 5.1 and 5.2 were obtained from patients who received majority of their treatments under my direction. The responses to the treatment were determined clinically as well as radiographically by independent radiologists. The recurrence-free survival in early stage breast cancer was determined by the time from diagnosis to the last time patient was known to be cancer-free. The survival time of patients with metastatic breast cancer was determined by the time from diagnosis to the last time patient is known to be alive. Kaplan-Meier's analysis was used for estimating the overall survival and progression-free survival during the study period.

The data indicates the integrated treatment model discussed above can lead to excellent clinical outcomes in breast cancer patients. Specifically, the following conclusions can be drawn:

1. Integrated oncology treatment combining weekly metronomic chemotherapy with selected naturopathic medicine has resulted in excellent clinical outcomes in patients with both early- and late-stage breast cancer. Routine integration of selected antioxidants and vitamins into the weekly chemotherapy treatment plans does not adversely affect the survival of breast cancer patients based on this series.
2. Integrative breast cancer treatment discussed in this poster may be particularly beneficial for patients who strongly desire to integrate complementary and alternative medicine into their treatment plans.
3. Prospective study of integrative breast cancer treatment based on the current model of care is warranted.

Table 5.1. Clinical Outcomes of Patients with Early Stage Breast Cancer after Integrative Therapy

	Median F/U(y)	Distand Relapse	Local Relapse	Relapse-Free Survival	Survival (NCDB*)
Stage I (14)	4	1 (7.4%)	0 (0%)	92.60%	100% (92)
Stage IIA (22)	6	0 (0%)	0 (0%)	100%	100% (81)
IIB (12)	6	1 (9%)	1 (9%)	82%	100% (74)
Stage IIIA (11)	6	2 (18%)	1 (9%)	73%	100% (67)
IIIB (7)	4	1 (14%)	3 (43%)	43%	86% (49)
IIIC (9)	5	0 (0%)	0 (0%)	100%	100% (49)

Table 5.2.   Clinical Outcomes of Advanced Stage Breast Cancer

Overall response rate	89%
Complete response	43%
Partial response	46%
Mixed response	11%
Progression-free survival (PFS)	1.2 years
5-year survival	53%
Median overall survival	5.8 years

LYMPHOMA STATISTICS

High-dose vitamin C in cancer treatment has been controversial. Although clinical trials with oral high-dose vitamin C in advanced cancer patients from the 1970s did not show any benefits in patients' survival,[7] more recent studies found intravenous high-dose vitamin C has different pharmacokinetics and anticancer effects. It was reported that high-dose intravenous vitamin C appears to generate hydrogen peroxide selectively in tumor tissues and causes oxidative damages to cancer cells but has little toxicity to normal cells.[8] In small clinical trials high-dose intravenous vitamin C reduced the side effects of chemotherapy in ovarian cancer patients with no negative impact on treatment outcomes. Based on laboratory studies, lymphoma may be one of the most susceptible malignancies to the biological effect of high-dose intravenous vitamin C.[9]

We conducted a retrospective review of medical records of thirty-six patients with various forms of non-Hodgkin's lymphoma including indolent lymphomas, diffuse large cell lymphoma, mantle cell lymphoma treated with conventional chemotherapy as well as high-dose intravenous vitamin C in an integrative setting at our cancer treatment center.

Patients responded very favorably to this combined treatment approach. Nearly all patients treated in the front-line setting responded to the treatment and achieved long progression-free survival and overall survival. Several patients with very aggressive forms of lymphomas achieved complete remission that have not recurred after long-term follow-up. All patients have tolerated high-dose vitamin C infusions with minimal side effects.

It can be concluded that high-dose intravenous vitamin C in conjunction with conventional chemotherapy can lead to excellent clinical out-

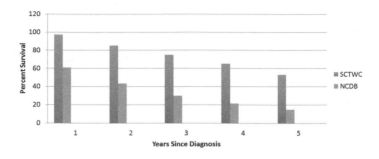

Figure 5.1.   Observed 5-Year Survival of Patients with Stage IV Breast Cancer

comes in patients with non-Hodgkin's lymphoma with minimal added side effects. In addition to the cases of lymphoma refractory to convention treatments, these cases strongly support the integration of high-dose intravenous vitamin C into all lymphoma treatment regimens. Further controlled clinical trials are warranted.

High-dose vitamin C has been widely used as a complementary cancer therapy. Increasing evidence suggests that high-dose intravenous vitamin C functions as a prodrug for hydrogen peroxide that induces cell death through oxidation-induced cell damage rather that apoptosis. This effect is relatively selective in tumor tissues due to its lack of catalase enzyme that degrades H2O2.[10] The hypoxic environment of tumor may also enhance the influx of vitamin C into tumor cells via hypoxia-induced factor (HIF). Additionally, tumor cells have relatively low antioxidant levels and are more susceptible to the pro-oxidative effect of high-dose vitamin C. Anecdotal reports of lymphoma remission due to high-dose vitamin C ignited the initial interest in using high-dose vitamin C in the treatment of cancer. Subsequently, various in vitro studies have demonstrated cytotoxicity of high-dose vitamin C against multiple tumor cell lines, especially lymphoma. At our center, cancer patients are co-managed by oncologists and naturopathic physicians trained in oncology who have commonly used high-dose vitamin C in the supportive cancer care. Here we report that these patients have achieved excellent clinical outcomes.

From Tables 5.3 and 5.4, the following conclusions can be drawn:

1. Concurrent administration of high-dose intravenous vitamin C with bio-chemotherapy in the treatment of indolent and aggressive non-Hodgkin's lymphomas resulted in excellent clinical responses.

Table 5.3.   Treatment Outcomes of Indolent Non-Hodgkin's Lymphoma Combining Chemotherapy and HDC

Median age	52
Dx: FL MZL LPL	7
	4
	1
Stage III–IV	5
	7
Median f/u	
Response CR/nCR PR	100%
	92% (11)
	8% (1)
PFS (months)	44
OS (months)	Not reached
Response CR/nCR PR	100%
	92% (11)
	8% (1)

2. Concurrent and maintenance administration of high-dose intravenous vitamin C were associated with prolonged progression-free survival of some indolent lymphoma patients, suggesting that high-dose vitamin C may alter the natural course of indolent lymphomas.

3. Concurrent and maintenance administration of high-dose vitamin C was associated with dramatic long-term survival in some patients with aggressive lymphoma that usually has poor prognosis.

4. High-dose vitamin C infusion has been very well tolerated with only rare infusional reactions.

These data sets are not from rigorous clinical trials, and for that, we may be criticized. Although a reductionist-style trial is necessary for confirming the benefits of many individual treatment modalities, a model of care like ours needs to be looked at as whole and outcome data evaluated against common statistics outside of our model. This is the work in progress at our center, and when the analysis is complete, we will show the results to the world. To our patients, whatever has worked for them is what really counts.

Table 5.4. Treatment Outcomes of Diffuse Large B Cell and Mantle Cell Lymphoma Combining Chemotherapy and HDC

Median age	50
Dx: DLBCL MCL	
	6
	6
Stage I–II	2
Stage III–IV	10
Median f/u	
Response CR/nCR PR	100%
	100% (12)
	0%
PFS (months)	Not reached
OS (months)	Not reached

6

MOVING FORWARD WITH INTEGRATIVE CANCER TREATMENT

In recent years, oncology has witnessed new developments that have the potential to disrupt the field. These are targeted therapy or precision medicine and immunotherapy. How does integrated therapy work with these new modalities of cancer treatment? Since our treatment model is multi-targeted and addresses the fundamental issues of cancer development and treatment, it can serve as a strong base on which to add these new therapies for further improvement of treatment outcomes.

PRECISION MEDICINE

The last decade in oncology has been marked by rapid unmasking of cancer genome and understanding of the molecular mechanisms of cancer development and progression. The technology of rapid DNA sequencing has made it possible to quickly identify specific DNA mutations that may serve as the "driver" of cancer growth. [1]

The remarkable progress in DNA sequencing technology has led to the identification of increasing numbers of common mutant genes in patients with different types of cancers. The accumulated data has led scientists to speculate that all cancers are more appropriately subclassified based on their genetic traits rather than their tissue origin. Drugs targeting these mutations have generated dramatic responses in certain subtypes of cancers, such as lung cancers that carry unique mutations such as EGFR mutation,[2] but only mediocre results in most other solid tumors. Additionally, patients who have targetable mutations are still a small minority of the overall patient population. As our knowledge of cancer molecular biology deepens in the near future, more and more single and combined targeted therapy options will emerge and bring about good treatment responses from more types of cancer.

However, the limitations of this cancer treatment approach are also obvious. First, cancer cells are highly unstable in their genetic structures and their DNA will remain a moving target for targeted therapy drugs. Second, since cancers have many alternative biochemical pathways, targeting one of them may only lead to their partial reduction or a slowdown of growth. This sets the stage for surviving cancer cells to become resistant. Thirdly, these targeted drugs are not always 100 percent specific for their targets, which leads to side effects that are sometimes more severe than chemotherapy.

Previous efforts to add maximum tolerated dosing (MTD) chemotherapy to targeted therapy did not show any significant benefits in the case of lung cancer.[3] This may be because the negative interaction of MTD chemo with the targeted therapy agents. Since targeted drugs often put cancer cells to sleep in a dormant state, it may affect chemotherapy effectiveness. However, targeted therapy may work well with the multitargeted MLDC, which does not depend so much on the cell replication to exert its function.[4] Targeted therapy is also a good choice as a maintenance therapy after the patient has had a good response to MLDC to prevent cancer cell reactivation and to prolong the patient's time without cancer progression. As these drugs generally have less or different side effects than chemotherapy, they can also provide patients a good respite after chemotherapy to avoid its accumulative side effects.

The story of patient Ellen discussed in chapter 5 is a good example of using targeted therapy drug Tarceva to maintain a long-lasting remission following her effective metronomic chemotherapy treatment. Future studies will need to look at optimal combinations of metronomic chemotherapy with various targeted therapy drugs to explore their synergy. Integrative therapies that boost the immune response and decrease inflammation can also help improve the efficacy of targeted therapy drugs and to reduce their potential side effects.

IMMUNOTHERAPY

As an integrative oncologist I have always advocated the importance of the immune system in cancer control. However, I have also encountered suspicion, if not outright ridicule, by some of my colleagues for many years.

The immune system? Does it do anything? Forget about it!

However, over the past few years immunotherapy has become a buzzword in the cancer community, and even among the general public, due to the rapid development of drugs that have produced some eye-opening results in several types of cancers that used to be particularly hard to treat with conventional therapies. Now everyone thinks that immunotherapy is our biggest hope to overcome cancer someday. Immunotherapy centers are being established inside cancer hospitals and clinics around the country to administer these treatments that are based on activating the immune system—just another confirmation that we live in a drug-happy world.

Although these immunotherapeutic drugs are certainly powerful, and their development is a step in the right direction, they are just another tool that we have in our toolbox to address the cancer problem. Just like any other drug that once generated the hope of conquering cancer, immunotherapeutic drugs are not the magic bullet that will shoot down cancer once and for all. Imparting the integrative approaches we have discussed in this book to the general cancer community will not only improve the odds of controlling cancer, it will also improve the quality of life of cancer patients, a goal of equal importance.

Immunotherapy is not a new concept. In the history of medicine there are several reports of deliberately infecting a tumor to suppress tumor progression. William Coley, a New York surgeon in the late nineteenth century, considered by some to be the father of modern cancer immunotherapy, tried to induce an anticancer immune response by injecting patients with bacterial toxins. Coley's vaccine, combining two virulent bacteria *Stretococcus pyrogens* and *Serratia marceacens*, was used to treat various cancer patients. Although the benefits of Coley's vaccine have never been proven by formal studies, it marked the first attempt to systematically use the immune system to fight cancer.

For several decades, Dr. Stephen Rosenberg, from the National Cancer Institute, has been conducting research on adoptive T cell transfer for treating cancer. His methods mainly involve isolating T cells from excised tumor tissues and expanding them with cytokines, before reinfusing them back into patients. Variable success has been seen in the treatment of melanoma and several other cancers. It was found that the efficacy of this method was dependent on how much the tumor had already been infiltrated by immune T cells before the treatment.[5]

In the early 1990s, the concept of checkpoint inhibitors was first proposed. Several molecules on the surface of T cells, including PD-1 and CTLA-4, were found to play an important role in the suppression of T-cell immune responses. Engagement of these receptors by ligands on the surface of the tumor cell led to "exhaustion" and eventual "suicide" of the affected T cells. Blocking these receptors was proposed as a mechanism to prevent cancer cells from suppressing T cells.[6]

The first commercial success came in 2011 when the FDA approved ipilimumab (Yervoy), a monoclonal antibody against CTLA4, in the treatment of melanoma. In a large randomized study, ipilimumab increased one-year survival rates from 25 percent to 46 percent, and two-year survival rates from 14 percent to 23 percent in patients with advanced melanoma when compared to controls.[7]

Ipilimumab became the first in a class of immune checkpoint inhibitors that "took the brakes off immune T cells," thereby activating them to fight cancer. It is often associated with severe but manageable side effects similar to autoimmune attacks on various organs and tissues.

The company that developed Yervoy moved on quickly to develop another checkpoint inhibitor, nivolumab (Opdivo). This is a monoclonal antibody that binds to PD-1 molecules on T cell surfaces, disrupting its interaction with its ligand PDL-1 on tumor cell surfaces. In patients with advanced non-small cell lung cancer that worsened after initial chemotherapy, 20 percent showed shrinkage of the tumor compared to 9 percent with docetaxel chemotherapy, the control arm. Importantly, 16 percent of Opdivo-treated patients were still alive after five years with no progression of the disease, suggesting the development of long-lasting tumor immunity. The expected five-year survival rate for the non-small cell lung cancer patients receiving continuous conventional treatment is only 4 percent.[8] Since then multiple other checkpoint inhibitors have been approved by FDA to treat cancers including melanoma, lung cancer, head and neck cancer, renal cancer, bladder cancer, and Hodgkin's lymphoma.

As you can see, the efficacy of these checkpoint inhibitors is still fairly limited, inducing a response in these treated patients no more than 30 percent of the time. It has been found that a tumor response to these checkpoint inhibitors depends on several factors. One is the level of expression of PD1 ligand PDL-1 on the surface of the tumor cells.[9] The benefits of this treatment are directly proportional to the level of PDL-1 expression. Another factor is the degree of tumor tissue T-cell infiltration before the treatment. A lack of T cells in tumor tissues, called "cold tumor," is usually an indicator of poor predicted response to checkpoint inhibitors. Another factor that can affect the response to these immunotherapies is the presence of immune suppressive cells such as Treg cells and MDSC.[10]

Metronomic chemotherapy can positively influence all of these factors associated with poor response to checkpoint inhibitor therapy. MLDC has been shown to increase the T-cell entry into tumor tissues (turning a cold tumor to a hot tumor) and improve immune response by suppressing MDSC and Treg cells. MDSC is known to prevent T-cell entry into tumor tissues. In this setting, integrative therapies are also required to maintain the healthfulness of immune T cells so that they can have good functions after activation. Lack of vital nutrients and exercise, depression and general systemic inflammation can all dampen the T-cell response even after they are released from the tumor-induced suppression. Therefore, the future for MLDC and integrative therapies are now becoming brighter and more important as more immunotherapy drugs are being used for all different kinds of cancer treatment.

Another very promising form of immunotherapy is called CAR T (Chimeric Antigen Receptor T cell) therapy.[11] It is a form of gene therapy that engineers T cells from cancer patients to recognize a unique target on cancer cell surface and expand them to large numbers before infusing back to the patients. This approach has found significant success in treating liquid tumors or hematological malignancies like acute lymphoblastic leukemia or multiple myeloma, since these tumor cells are easily killed by the CAR T cells in the blood or bone marrow. However, there has not been real success of this treatment for solid tumors, probably because of the difficulty of tumor penetration by these T cells or preexisting immune suppressive mechanisms in these tumors. In the future, MLDC may be used to open up the solid tumor and expose their antigens before patients are given back the reengineered T cells to decrease suppressor cell function and to enhance CAR T cell tumor penetration.

OUR CURRENT CHALLENGE

Recall that someone is diagnosed with cancer in America every twenty-three seconds. The American Cancer Society estimates that nearly 2 million *new* patients will need treatment in 2018. Judging from current trends and treatment methods, far too many of these people will be treated *without* the benefits of an integrated treatment protocol. This means their immune systems will not be properly cared for, thus making the effects of high-dose chemotherapy even more dangerous. The same risks also apply to the new treatment modalities. If we continue to focus exclusively on a single form of cancer therapy and not an integrative plan addressing multiple aspects of the cancer, we likely will still not get very far because cancer is just not a simple disease that can be taken down with a single bullet, no matter how magical it may be.

However, in our drug happy culture, it is very easy for people to get overexcited about a single seemingly perfect treatment and forget the comprehensive needs of our whole body. We need more education and promotion of holistic concept of cancer care to make real and sustained improvement of cancer treatment outcomes. Moreover, as much research as possible should be conducted to validate the perceived value of many integrated therapies, even though they may appear obvious and self-evident. This will help convince the general medical community not already familiar with the integrative concept and will serve as a foundation for further development of these treatment modalities.

CASE REPORT

Rozlyn is a mellow, easygoing, and well-humored lady in her sixties who suddenly came down with a seizure. She was found to have at least two cancerous lesions on parts of her brain, and further whole-body CT scans showed that these cancerous brain lesions came from a large tumor on her left upper lung, with multiple satellite lesions and enlarged lymph nodes in the middle of her chest. She underwent emergent craniotomies to remove these two lesions form her brain, which confirmed that the brain tumor came from metastatic lung cancer.

She was initially treated with conventional systemic chemotherapy. She experienced transient response for a couple of months, then cancer started to enlarge again relentlessly. She was then told by her oncologist to get her affairs in order. When she came to see me, I started her on salvage therapy with the newly available immunotherapy nivolumab (Opdivo). To improve her chance of response and long-term remission, I also started her on oral metronomic low-dose chemotherapy with cyclophosphamide. She tolerated both treatments well, and in three months her cancer diminished in activity. After six months, her cancer went into complete remission as determined by a PET-CT scan. She also had no new or residual brain metastasis. She is now three years from her diagnosis and has remained in remission for almost two years. She had recently enjoyed traveling with her husband in an RV from Seattle to Branson, Missouri, for a family reunion. Rozlyn's case illustrates that even in the most severe cases of cancer now there is hope in the new treatment modality combining immunotherapy with metronomic chemotherapy.

Laura is a seventy-two-year-old woman who enjoys playing piano in a quartet with her two brothers and a sister. She was diagnosed with recurrent ER/PR positive HER-2/Neu negative breast cancer metastasized to her liver and bones about seven years ago. For the first three years after diagnosis, she was given one anti-estrogen therapy after another but eventually progressed on every one of them. Symptoms of cancer involving bones and liver also started to emerge. At that time, she started seeing me, and over the next four years she rotated through sixteen different chemotherapy drugs given sequentially or in combination by metronomic dosing.

Laura's cancer mostly remained under control until about a year ago, when her CA27.29 started to go up very fast along with rapid increase in sizes and numbers of tumor in her liver. She received treatment with CyberKnife to control several rapidly growing liver lesions and tumor marker CA27.29 decreased transiently for several weeks, then spiked again. At that time she was placed in a compassionate use program to receive the immunotherapy drug nivolumab (Opdivo), initially with oral cyclophosphamide, but the cancer marker continued to increase rapidly, and she started to show signs of liver failure with development of large ascites as well as severe leg edema.

She was switched to combination metronomic chemotherapy with weekly epirubicine, cyclophosphamide, leucovorin, and 5-Fu, while continuing immunotherapy with nivolumab. Within three to four weeks her ascites and leg fluid retention almost completely resolved. Her liver enzymes returned to normal range. Everyone could see that her health condition had had another dramatic turnaround. As of this writing, Laura has received three months of combined MLDC and immunotherapy with nivolumab, and is overall doing very well. Her tumor marker has dropped over 70 percent and is close to baseline.

Laura's case illustrates that combination MLDC can enhance the efficacy of new immunotherapy drugs to induce major improvement in cancer control, even in a very advanced condition. This is consistent with the mechanisms of action of MLDC in augmenting antitumor immune response and to inducing immunogenic tumor cell death.

OFFERING GENUINE HOPE

We have seen that cancer does not have to be a death sentence, and that treating it does not have to kill any more of the patient than the cancer is already doing. With advances in immunotherapy and integrated therapy, it is entirely reasonable to expect that cancer can become a chronic disease or, in many cases, cured by an integrative treatment and changes in general lifestyle.

This speaks directly to the main purpose of this book, which is to let patients know about treatment options that may not be discussed at conventional cancer centers, since most people are just following protocols and are not encouraged to think out of the box. It's OK when there are relatively good conventional treatment options, but if you are diagnosed with cancer and do not have very good options, it pays to look more broadly for options that have both a good science base and clinical experience, even though that may not be the current standard of practice. Simply put, if you have a cancer that is known to have a poor prognosis based on conventional care and you just look at the conventional treatment alone, you will get just that. At minimum, you should think about integrating complementary supportive measures for all the good reasons we discussed here. Newly diagnosed patients and those whose current treatment is ineffective are both potential beneficiaries of integrative treatments.

A secondary reason for this book, but one ultimately as valuable, is to inform oncologists and expand the conversation about the success of treatments integrating MLDC and complementary medicine. Our hope is that patients and those taking care of them will discover the value of this comprehensive umbrella of integrative therapies and begin using them correctly to obtain better results.

We have extremists on both sides who create polarized situations with their stubborn viewpoints—for example, that MTD is the only way to go or that any drug is bad and should be avoided at all cost. Neither of these positions will do anyone any good. Consider the case of someone diagnosed with heart disease. A cardiologist does not say, "I'm going to cure you," because we don't *cure* heart disease once and for all, end of story. We also don't cure diabetes or most chronic, degenerative diseases. We *manage* them.

What should we tell patients with stage 4 cancer? "You're going to die"? "You have only so many months to live"? "Get your affairs in order"? Based only on common statistics, oncologists routinely deliver these prognostications to their patients—and in such an authoritative manner that, to patients, they sound like the word of God or of someone with a big crystal ball. Of course, there is nothing wrong in disclosing the statistics of a certain cancer. However, please do make it clear that these are just statistics and may not represent the individual patient who may fall on any point in the statistical range. Encourage your patient to participate in his or her own care and consider all beneficial treatment options so that he or she can move up on the statistical range and achieve better-than-average survival. It is very true—and I see it all the time—that hope is the main supporting pillar of a patient's life. Someone with hope usually has a much better chance of surviving even in the face of an aggressive cancer; whereas someone who has lost hope tends to die prematurely. Therefore, when engaging in "straight talk" with your patients, don't take away their hope for recovery and become a disservice to them. In my practice, I find one of the benefits of integrative care is the hope it instills in patients that they can get better, with our help, through their own actions. Diet, nutrition, exercise, and early signs of treatment response all become positive reinforcements that grow stronger over time and become therapeutic themselves.

We believe in promoting hope, not despair.

CHANGING OUR BELIEF SYSTEM

We have many patients in our practice with stage 4 cancers who are alive and well, five, ten, or more years after they were told they had no hope. Among them are patients with pancreatic, lung, colon, bladder, breast, and ovarian cancers, as well as lymphoma and soft tissue sarcoma. Some of these patients even had cancers involving the brain. Many have seen their cancers come completely under control; they remain only on a maintenance or a monitoring program. Despite statistical caveats, I strongly believe that we can stack our numbers against any national or institutional averages in the country. It's not that we are doing any magic or creating secret recipes; we are just using a more commonsense approach that has been reinforced by steady and consistent successes. So how can we help change the conventional oncology world to help patients better? I've always felt it is a belief system that is at the core of the human problem. So, let's start asking the question around the table: Do you still believe that medicine is both an art and a science? My answer is definitely a yes!

As oncologists, we are constantly being bombarded by a myriad of new information from pharmaceutical industries and academic opinion leaders on how we should treat our patients, but have we thought often enough or at all to ask our patients how they want to be treated? After all, we are dealing with living, thinking, feeling individuals, not just machines that need to be fixed. If you still don't believe in the value of integrative care, put yourself in the shoes of your patients and ask yourself the following question: As human beings, our systems are sophisticated and integrated. We all need to eat better, sleep better, exercise more, fortify our food with nutrients when we need them, and, above all, we all need HOPE to live. *Why the exception in the diagnosis of cancer?*

Realizing the obvious answer to this question, it's time to really study the needs of our patients and to support them as whole persons. We also need to be very mindful of treatments that disrupt the balances of these life forces and ask ourselves how we can do better. In this world of oncology dominated by doctrines and commercial interests, it is understandably difficult to have any original thinking. But for the sake of our patients, and to honor our Hippocratic oaths, we need to. If you open your mind's eye, embrace your inner scientist, and eschew any preset dogma, you will see that what I have described in this book is not only reasonable but also well supported by science. Our approach centers on fostering and augmenting the immune system with MLDC and integrative therapies. It starts out with a gentler, steadier approach to cancer control while empowering our patients with concrete plans to support them both body and soul. The goal is to gradually shift the balance of power between the immune system and the cancer in their bodies to their favor. It is a slow and laborious process not without significant challenges. However, it is also a process with the power of self-reinforcement. As the confidence builds with each small success, the hope becomes an increasingly powerful ally in our fight against cancer.

So, as a healthcare provider, how can I serve my patients better? This is my constant challenge and a question I ask myself every day. We never tell our patients that we have all the answers; no one does. But we do let them know that we are on this ride *with them* and we listen carefully to their voices. In this crazy world of sound bites and sales pitches, oncology has its own four-letter word: *hope*. In the Greek myth of Pandora's Box, it is often forgotten that after everything negative inside was unleashed, something special remained at the bottom: HOPE!

Hope is the antidote. If you let hope lapse, there's not a lot you can do regardless of your genius. However, fostering hope in the place of despair takes both heart and wisdom. The idea of this book is to give patients, as well as their doctors, the courage, information, and inspiration to work together and find the most sensible and comprehensive solutions to the problems of cancer.

Here is the chance, for patients and doctors, to follow a new path, one that has been around for a long, long time. Here is the chance to try, because if nobody tries, nothing better will happen. This is the essence of *Rx for Hope*.

Q & A

With Dr. Nick Chen

NOTE: The following questions and answers provide a capsulated over-view of the work Dr. Nick Chen is doing at the Seattle Integrative Cancer Center in Seattle, Washington.

1. How do you see the current climate of cancer care in America?

Conventional treatment is still dominated by outdated methods using maximum tolerated doses of chemotherapy, which causes toxic effects both seen and unseen, such as fatigue, nausea, malnutrition, infection, systemic inflammation, and immunosuppression. While most cancer patients are still relying on this fairly ineffective and toxic form of cancer treatment for the foreseeable future, most oncology researchers are solely focusing on the molecular structures of cancer, trying to find its "Achilles tendon" and a magic-bullet-like pill to cure it. Without taking note of the microenvironment the cancer actually grows in, this approach is akin to "seeing the tree but missing the forest," and its impact on the overall cancer control will be slow and limited. With the pharmaceutical industry dominating the scene, the emphasis on cancer treatment leans too much toward drug development rather than toward improving our basic approach to cancer care, such as improving the way of delivering chemotherapy and providing complementary supportive care for cancer patients. This has created a void of important knowledge about taking care of a patient as a whole person and most patients still don't have the benefit of an integrative approach in their cancer care plan that emphasizes the importance of diet, nutrition, supplements, exercise, and other wellness measures, to support the essential cancer control immune system.

As a society, we have so much pessimism toward cancer that we are often readier to give up on a cancer patient than to think creatively to help him or her get through it. We are bound by so many societal doctrines and insurance policies aimed at resource utilization that physicians just don't have much independence in medical decision-making or to think outside of the box or to go extra miles to help our patients. It seems that we may have forgotten that we are dealing with human lives, and not machines that are just running on preset codes. It seems that commercial interests and even politics, rather than the true interests of cancer patients, are dominating the scene of cancer care sometimes.

2. How does this approach affect you as an oncologist?

Oncologists today have to prescribe drug therapies for their patients that are also toxic, which directly hampers their ability to fight cancer. They have few tools at their disposal to balance these negative effects. Yes, we have fairly effective medicine for preventing or treating chemo-induced nausea, but how about correcting malnutrition, improving a patient's sense of well-being, and most importantly, reversing the immunosuppression that is caused by the cancer in the first place, and then worsened by the treatment?

There are no satisfactory answers for these questions in conventional guidelines, and as a result, most oncologists either think these issues are not important or they just don't know what to do. When an integrative oncology practice like ours tries to be mindful about the defects in the current treatment methodology—leading us to adjust our treatment strategy and by integrating various supportive measures based on science and commons sense—we are sometimes looked upon differently or suspiciously by conventional cancer communities.

3. How do you see patients being affected by this situation?

Patients are missing the opportunity to optimize their odds of getting over cancer and bettering their quality of life along the way. Doctors are missing the chance to be a part of making this happen!

4. How do these issues apply specifically to chemotherapy treatment?

By definition, current cytotoxic chemotherapy treatment using maximal tolerated doses causes many toxicities, both seen and unseen, such as fatigue, nausea, malnutrition, neutropenic infections, systemic inflammation, and immunosuppression. We need to fundamentally change this by giving more low-dose and regular chemo treatments that are in general less toxic and more consistent in their capacity to suppress cancer.

However, oncology researchers are increasingly becoming extensions of pharmaceutical industries that are looking for new and more profitable drugs. Therefore, little interest and effort are being put into improving the paradigm of basic cancer treatment methods, that is, the traditional chemotherapy methods and its supportive care.

5. What is a "commonsense approach" to cancer care?

This refers to an approach of cancer care taken from the understanding that our inner healing power, the immune system, holds the key to ultimate cancer control and the immune system can be supported by simple changes in our lifestyles and nutrition. This represents a paradigm shift in the way cancer has traditionally been treated, which mostly relies on using high doses of drugs to kill cancer cells.

6. How do you optimize a patient's immune system for long-term cancer survival?

First, we must do no harm and limit the impact of cytotoxic chemotherapy drugs. We know we can achieve better cancer control by using metronomic low-dose chemotherapy. Second, we must enhance patients' immune systems as part of the cancer treatment using integrative therapies. These include measures such as diet, nutrition, exercise, selective supplements, mind-body therapy, and whatever support that can be beneficial for proper immune system function. Thirdly, we would use the newest immunotherapy agents such as checkpoint inhibitors to give overall immune supportive therapy a boost. The goal is to turn cancer into a chronic disease controlled by the patient's own immune system.

7. Does science support the idea of a mind/body connection affecting our health?

Clinical studies around the world have repeatedly shown that our state of mind can strongly influence our immune system and the outcomes of cancer treatment. The scientific basis for this connection comes through the relatively new discipline of psychoneuroimmunology, which has established a crucial link between prominent neurotransmitters in our brain and our immune system.

For example, multiple studies indicate that depression is associated with higher mortality even after controlling for stages of disease and levels of patient participation in their treatments.[1] In the California Breast Cancer Study, women with the most suppressed emotions had a four-fold increase of mortality after diagnosis. In a twelve-year follow-up study conducted by the University of Rochester and Harvard Medical School of Public Health, people with the most suppressed emotions had a 70 percent increased risk of developing cancer during the study period. In a University of Miami study, men with suppressed emotions were found to have significantly decreased NK cell numbers and activity, both of which are important for controlling the progression of cancer.[2]

While positive mind activities, such as relaxation and encouragement, increase the brain's production of endorphins, which is known to directly stimulate immune system cells like T-lymphocytes and NK cells, negative emotions, such as depression, anxiety, and stress, can lead to a decrease in endorphin production. This indicates that when it comes to cancer prevention and control, we can see a crucial connection between our brain and immune function.

8. Why don't most oncologists recognize this science?

The general shortage of attention paid to the role of the mind and body in cancer care is partly due to a lack of understanding of the importance of the immune system in controlling cancer and how much it is affected by mind/body interactions. This not only affects a patient's treatment outcome; it is also a determining factor during the entire cancer journey and the patient's quality of life after the initial diagnosis.

This can also be partly blamed on Western medical education that focuses almost entirely on pharmaceutical and physical interventions in disease treatment. Without a holistic view of disease, this process leads to a medical system that emphasizes the treatment of a specific disease without changing the physical and physiological environments that may cause the disease in the first place.

9. What is metronomic low-dose chemotherapy and what are its benefits?

Metronomic low-dose chemotherapy, which is a major part of our treatment program, uses traditional medicine to treat cancer given more regularly and in lower doses. This makes the treatment more tolerable and effective. It is based on giving just enough chemotherapy and hitting cancer cells at the right time and without letting them recover between treatment cycles.

Through novel mechanisms, including antiangiogenesis and immune modulation, this treatment methodology can create long-lasting cancer control in many patients while maintaining quality of life, as evidenced by the many successful stories from patients throughout this book.

Another advantage of low-dose chemotherapy is that it synergizes with rather than counteracting the benefits of complementary and supportive therapies that aim to improve a patient's immune system and nutritional status. When all the treatments work together, patients benefit the most.

10. Is there a financial incentive for pharmas to support low-dose chemo?

With drugs that are still under patent protection, pharma companies may be interested in sponsoring studies of their drugs that can be given in a more effective and less toxic way, which should increase their use by cancer patients and be good for a company's profits. However, most times metronomic regimes use cheap generic drugs that no pharma companies are incentivized to support their studies anymore.

11. Describe naturopathic medicine and what role it plays in your practice?

First of all, naturopathy is not "alternative" medicine. More and more it is becoming appropriately referred to as complementary, a holistic system of medicine based on the well-researched, healing power of nature, which has been practiced around the globe since our origins. In every culture, indigenous medicine uses diet, plants, nutrients, and naturally derived substances (nutraceuticals) to help heal the body, mind, and spirit of an individual. This is the foundation of our approach, to support our patients as people and respect their inner power to heal.

In our clinic, naturopathy consultations guide patients with their diet, nutrition, and lifestyle, along with judicious use of nutritional supplements to help boost the immune system and to reduce the side effects of conventional treatment.

We are combining these elements because we want to bring together the best of all sciences. When we engage patients in their own care, which naturopathy invites them to do, it allows for better, more substantial healing. Considering this, naturopathy plays an integral role in our patient care—on physical, emotional, and psychological levels.

12. What about medical marijuana?

It can play a supportive role during cancer treatment. Some of my patients have found it helpful for nausea, anorexia, and pain. Science has pointed to its potential benefit in cancer control. One problem we have is the variability and inconsistency of the preparations.

13. You treat many patients with stage 4 cancers. How do they fare with you?

The dogma in today's medical oncology world remains—if you have most forms of stage 4 cancer, you can't be cured and you're going to die, usually, according to the status quo based on conventional MTD treatments, within a few months to a few years. This means that the goal of mainstream oncology treatment is just to extend life or palliate cancer symptoms. Sometimes patients with advanced cancer are treated with a couple of conventional protocols and are told that they had run out of options and should get their affairs in order.

We have consistently seen very positive results with stage 4 patients such as those with lung, breast, colon, ovarian, bladder, prostate, or even pancreatic cancers, many of whom have been with us for five, ten, or even more years. Although I don't think any of them are really cured, I believe a simple change in how we deliver chemotherapy and integration of complementary therapies have made all the difference in the survival of these patients by turning some of their cancers into chronic rather than immediately life-threatening diseases.

14. Does the medical establishment need an attitude adjustment?

Our society harbors a historical pessimism toward cancer. Unfortunately, the medical establishment reinforces that psychology whenever they opt to give up on a patient rather than think creatively to find a solution. The oncology field is bound by guidelines that do not easily support innovation and policies that do not encourage doctors to think outside of the box. This can result in overlooking the deeply human element, that people are not machines and their health cannot always be determined by data and preset codes.

While oncologists continue to think they have to prescribe treatments that are highly toxic and actually hamper a patient's ability to fight cancer, they have few tools at their disposal to balance these negative effects, let alone build up the patient's ability to ultimately thrive—during and after treatment. We have fairly effective medicine for preventing or treating chemo-induced nausea and other temporary side effects, but how about correcting malnutrition, improving a patient's sense of well-being, and most important, reversing immunosuppression caused by the cancer and the treatment?

Conventional guidelines offer no answers to this question. As a result, oncologists either consider these issues unimportant or they just don't know what to do about them. An integrative oncology practice like ours tries to be mindful about the defects in this methodology. We adjust our treatment strategy while integrating various supportive measures that are based on both science and common sense.

Unfortunately, conventional cancer communities, for the most part, are still ignoring the value of integrative cancer care. This is sad and often frustrating because patients and their doctors are missing opportunities to optimize their odds of surviving cancer and improving their general health along the way.

15. What is your prognosis for cancer care?

Considering my patients' experience in our integrated model of cancer treatment, I am hopeful. But if we just keep searching and hoping for a magic bullet to cure cancer we will probably be disappointed. This is because cancer is such a complex disease with its own survival mechanism that continues to adapt to drugs thrown at them. The odds improve significantly if we can motivate and guide our immune system to control the cancer. Human evolution has clearly demonstrated that our immune system is our most efficient and versatile weapon to fight off diseases like infection and cancer.

To achieve this, we must first do no harm—or as little as possible—to our immune systems, which means we should avoid maximally tolerated chemotherapy. Evidence shows that when we switch to metronomic low-dose chemotherapy we actually may enhance the anticancer immune response by rebalancing different immune cells with opposite functions. We should also utilize all tools of integrative medicine to boost our immune system so that it will eventually take control.

16. If you could deliver a lecture to oncologists and cancer executives at an ASCO [American Society of Clinical Oncology] gathering, what would you tell them about the current state of oncology in America?

Even with the rapid advances in cancer treatment through pharmaceutical research, oncology treatment is still not able to give most cancer patients a consistent treatment response while maintaining a good quality of life. For example, the initial response rate to treatment for advanced lung cancer is about 30 percent; for colon cancer it is 60 percent, and for breast cancer it is 65 percent, but the side effects from the treatments are universally associated with a decrease in the quality of life and an increase in treatment failure, both short and long term.

The current state of affairs in the world of oncology is due in large part to a fundamental defect in the basic way we approach cancer care. Chemotherapy regimens are still based on decades-old dogmas of maximally tolerated doses. If we ever want to see substantial improvement in cancer treatment outcomes, this needs to be overhauled. Metronomic low-dose chemotherapy is less toxic and more consistent in killing cancer cells. Through anti-angiogenesis and immune modulation, it also controls the microenvironment where cancer cells grow. All these factors can lead to significant improvements in treatment outcomes, both in extending life and preserving its quality.

As we develop more precisely targeted medicines, we shouldn't forget that cancer is a complex disease whose development is due to genetics, personal life choices, and a host of environmental factors. Its impact on patients is equally multifaceted, affecting their mental, physical, and social life. All these factors affect key functions of the immune system and increase the risk of cancer resistance to treatment. Since the immune system may be the ultimate determining factor in long-term cancer control, we need to optimize the functionality of the immune system to maximize our patients' odds of long-term survival.

Our experience at Seattle Integrative Cancer Center is consistent with this theory. While we need additional systemic studies and documentation in order to expand the use of this methodology, we have seen over fifteen-plus years that metronomic low-dose chemotherapy and complementary naturopathic medicine can provide many long-term controls of cancer. Our patients with advanced cancers who have survived against all odds are living proof of the success of this integrative model.

17. Can your center become a viable, accepted model for others across the country?

It definitely can and should. Our tremendous patient treatment outcomes are unmatched compared with conventional treatments and provide strong testimony to the value of integrating metronomic low-dose chemotherapy with immune-boosting naturopathic and mind/body medicine.

We need to systemically document our approaches and educate the conventional cancer community about our methods. This will take time, but once people see the results, I think they will probably never want to continue with the same treatment methods they are using today.

18. Why is this book important for patients and medical professionals?

It presents viable alternatives to high-dose immunosuppressive chemotherapy and expands the menu for treating patients as whole persons. Our integrative model of cancer care offers a gentler but more consistent approach, using direct anticancer treatments, such as metronomic low-dose chemotherapy combined with natural immune-boosting therapies. All of this is supported by consistent treatment outcomes, exemplified by the many success stories of patients described in this book.

This is meant to educate patients about options outside the traditional offerings they may be familiar with, as well as opening the minds of conventional oncologists who are willing to explore new ways to improve their patients' treatment outcomes, and their quality of life.

As more and more patients realize the foundational importance of a healthy immune system—both in preventing and navigating any type of cancer treatment—they are also seeking simple, clear information from medical experts as well as real-life stories from patients who are living proof of the benefits and success of this approach.

We hope that our model of integrative cancer treatment, blending traditional Western medicine and holistic methods, will inspire patients and the cancer community as a whole to embrace the vital importance of taking care of our immune system.

19. Can cancer ever be completely cured?

Normally we do not view it this way. But we find over and over, more and more, that our patients are reversing the trends of recurrence. When their immune system is properly built up, as we do on a regular basis, the recurrences become farther apart and less frequent. And when it does flare up, we do not look at it as a failure, but rather as something to manage and control, like a chronic disease. It is my observation that our patients previously treated in an integrative care model also have a better chance to reestablish cancer control after a relapse.

20. Why *Rx for Hope*?

As doctors, we treat human beings. When a patient is diagnosed with cancer, emotions are thrown for a loop, but at the same time the emotional life plays a big role in their eventual healing. Hope, of course, becomes a central factor for them and their loved ones. And unlike what some may believe, doctors are human beings too and although we rely on science each day, we also live with hope in our hearts.

In that spirit, this book is intended to offer hope to patients who may not be finding it elsewhere and for those newly diagnosed who are seeking a somewhat different and more hopeful approach. We also want to impress our colleagues in the cancer care community with the idea that hope is vital to caring for patients and hope can be found in a different approach to our cancer care, as exemplified by so many of our patients' success stories throughout this book.

NOTES

1. FROM MUSTARD GAS
TO MODERN MEDICINE

1. A. B. Weisse (1991), *Medical Odysseys: The Different and Sometimes Unexpected Pathways to Twentieth-Century Medical Discoveries* (New Brunswick, NJ: Rutgers University Press), p. 127.

2. P. Christa (2011), "The Birth of Chemotherapy at Yale," Bicentennial Lecture Series: Surgery Grand Round, *Yale Journal of Biology and Medicine* 84(2): 169–72.

3. V. DeVita and E. Chu (2008), "A History of Cancer Chemotherapy," *Cancer Research* 68(21): 8643–53.

4. M. C. Li et al. (1956), "Effect of Methotrexate Therapy upon Choriocarcinoma and Chorioadenoma," *Proceedings of the Society for Experimental Biology and Medicine* 93(2): 361–66.

5. E. Freireich (2002), "Special Article: Min Chiu Li—A Perspective in Cancer Therapy," *Clinical Cancer Research* 8(9): 2764–65.

6. B. Fisher et al. (1993), "Lumpectomy Compared with Lumpectomy and Radiation Therapy for the Treatment of Intraductal Breast Cancer," *New England Journal of Medicine* 328(22): 1581–86.

7. G. Bonadonna et al. (1995), "Adjuvant Cyclophosphamide, Methotrexate, and Fluorouracil in Node-Positive Breast Cancer—The Results of 20 Years of Follow-Up," *New England Journal of Medicine* 332(14): 901–6.

8. M. Heron et al. (2006), "Deaths: Final Data for 2006," *National Vital Statistics Reports* 57(14): 1–134.

9. Y. Cao and R. Langer (2008), "A Review of Judah Folkman's Remarkable Achievements in Biomedicine," *Proceedings of the National Academy of Sciences of the United States of America* 105(36): 13203–5.

10. J. S. Carter (2014), "Mitosis," http://biology.clc.uc.edu/courses/bio104/mitosis.htm.

11. S. Nussey and S. Whitehead (2001), *Endocrinology: An Integrated Approach (Oxford, UK: BIOS Scientific Publishers Limited).*

2. IN DEFENSE OF OUR HEALTH

1. L. L. Lanier (2015), "NKG2D Receptor and Its Ligands in Host Defense," *Cancer Immunology Research* 3(6): 575–82.

2. M. Arap et al. (2004), "Cell Surface Expression of the Stress Response Chaperone GRP78 Enables Tumor Targeting by Circulating Ligands," *Cancer Cell* 6(3): 275–84.

3. B. Pulendran and R. Ahmed (2006), "Review Translating Innate Immunity into Immunological Memory: Implications for Vaccine Development," *Cell* 124(4): 849–63.

4. G. Dunn et al. (2002), "Cancer Immunoediting: From Immunosurveillance to Tumor Escape," *Nature Immunology* 3(11): 991–98.

5. M. D. Vesely et al. (2010), "Natural Innate and Adaptive Immunity to Cancer," *Annual Review of Immunology* 29: 235–71.

6. D. Fu et al. (2015), "Metabolic Perturbation Sensitizes Human Breast Cancer to NK Cell-Mediated Cytotoxicity by Increasing the Expression of MHC Class I Chain-Related A/B," *OncoImmunology* 4(3): 1–10.

7. K. Imai et al. (2000), "Natural Cytotoxic Activity of Peripheral-Blood Lymphocytes and Cancer Incidence: An 11-Year Follow-Up Study of a General Population," *Lancet* 356(9244): 1795–99.

8. G. Jobin et al. (2017), "Association between Natural Killer Cell Activity and Colorectal Cancer in High-Risk Subjects Undergoing Colonoscopy," *Gastroenterology* 153(4): 980–87.

9. A. Bhatia and Y. Kumar (2011), "Cancer-Immune Equilibrium: Questions Unanswered," *Cancer Microenvironment* 4(2): 209–17.

10. K. W. Hulsewé et al. (1999), "Nutritional Depletion and Dietary Manipulation: Effects on the Immune Response," *World Journal of Surgery* 23(6): 536–44.

11. K. Ryungsa et al. (2016), "A Role for Peripheral Natural Killer (NK) Cell Activity in the Response to Neoadjuvant Chemotherapy in Patients with Breast Cancer," *Journal of Clinical Oncology* 34(15): e12073.

12. V. Chandan et al. (2015), "Natural Killer (NK) Cell Profiles in Blood and Tumour in Women with Large and Locally Advanced Breast Cancer (LLABC) and Their Contribution to a Pathological Complete Response (PCR) in the Tumour Following Neoadjuvant Chemotherapy (NAC): Differential Restoration of Blood Profiles by NAC and Surgery," *Journal of Translational Medicine* 13(1): 1–21.

13. K. Duck-Hee et al. (2009), "Significant Impairment in Immune Recovery Following Cancer Treatment," *Nursing Research* 58(2): 105–14.

3. LESS IS MORE

1. K. Gammon (2012), "Mathematical Modelling: Forecasting Cancer," *Nature* 491(7425): S66–S67.

2. R. Kerbel et al. (2002), "Continuous Low-Dose Anti-Angiogenic/Metronomic Chemotherapy: From the Research Laboratory into the Oncology Clinic," *Annals of Oncology* 13(1): 12–15.

3. H. Skipper et al. (1964), "Experimental Evaluation of Potential Anticancer Agents. XIII: On the Criteria and Kinetics Associated with 'Curability' of Experimental Leukemia," *Cancer Chemotherapy Reports* 35: 1–111.

4. R. Simon and L. Norton (2006), "The Norton–Simon Hypothesis: Designing More Effective and Less Toxic Chemotherapeutic Regimens," *Nature Clinical Practice Oncology* 3(8): 406–7.

5. M. Citron et al. (2003), "Randomized Trial of Dose-Dense versus Conventionally Scheduled and Sequential versus Concurrent Combination Chemotherapy as Postoperative Adjuvant Treatment of Node-Positive Primary Breast Cancer: First Report of Intergroup Trial C9741/Cancer and Leukemia Group B Trial 9741," *Journal of Clinical Oncology* 21(8): 1431–39.

6. A. Chung et al. (2012), "Differential Drug Class-Specific Metastatic Effects Following Treatment with a Panel of Angiogenesis Inhibitors," *The Journal of Pathology* 227(4): 404–16.

7. G. Klement et al. (2002), "Differences in Therapeutic Indexes of Combination Metronomic Chemotherapy and an Anti-VEGFR-2 Antibody in Multidrug-Resistant Human Breast Cancer Xenografts," *Clinical Cancer Research* 8(1): 221–32.

8. T. Browder et al. (2000), "Antiangiogenic Scheduling of Chemotherapy Improves Efficacy against Experimental Drug-Resistant Cancer," *Cancer Research* 60(7): 1878–86.

9. B. Sennino et al. (2009), "Correlative Dynamic Contrast MRI and Microscopic Assessments of Tumor Vascularity in RIP-Tag2 Transgenic Mice," *Magnetic Resonance in Medicine* 62(3): 616–25.

10. F. Bertolini (2003), "Maximum Tolerable Dose and Low-Dose Metronomic Chemotherapy Have Opposite Effects on the Mobilization and Viability of Circulating Endothelial Progenitor Cells," *Cancer Research* 63(15): 4342–46.

11. T. S. Chan et al. (2016), "Metronomic Chemotherapy Prevents Therapy-Induced Stromal Activation and Induction of Tumor-Initiating Cells," *Journal of Experimental Medicine* 213(13): 2967–88.

12. V. Xavier et al. (2007), "Deficient CD4+CD25high T Regulatory Cell Function in Patients with Active Systemic Lupus Erythematosus," *Journal of Immunology* 178(4): 2579–88.

13. W. Licun (2011), "Tumor Cell Repopulation between Cycles of Chemotherapy Is Inhibited by Regulatory T-Cell Depletion in a Murine Mesothelioma Model," *Journal of Thoracic Oncology* 6(9): 1578–86.

14. P. Vicari (2009), "Paclitaxel Reduces Regulatory T Cell Numbers and Inhibitory Function and Enhances the Antitumor Effects of the TLR9 Agonist PF-3512676 in the Mouse," *Cancer Immunology, Immunotherapy* 58(4): 615–28.

15. L. A. Emens et al. (2009), "Timed Sequential Treatment with Cyclophosphamide, Doxorubicin, and an Allogeneic Granulocyte-Macrophage Colony-Stimulating Factor–Secreting Breast Tumor Vaccine: A Chemotherapy Dose-Ranging Factorial Study of Safety and Immune Activation," *Journal of Clinical Oncology* 27(35): 5911–18.

16. W. L. Michele et al. (2010), "Conditional Regulatory T-Cell Depletion Releases Adaptive Immunity Preventing Carcinogenesis and Suppressing Established Tumor Growth," *Cancer Research* 70(20): 7800–09.

17. K. Amy (2016), "Tumor-Induced MDSC Act via Remote Control to Inhibit L-Selectin-Dependent Adaptive 2 Immunity in Lymph Nodes," *eLife* 5: e17375.

18. R. Vedran et al. (2010), "Cyclophosphamide Resets Dendritic Cell Homeostasis and Enhances Antitumor Immunity through Effects That Extend beyond Regulatory T Cell Elimination," *Cancer Immunology, Immunotherapy* 59(1): 137–48.

19. J. P. H. Machiels et al. (2001), "Cyclophosphamide, Doxorubicin, and Paclitaxel Enhance the Antitumor Immune Response of Granulocyte/Macrophage-Colony Stimulating Factor-Secreting Whole-Cell Vaccines in HER-2/Neu Tolerized Mice," *Cancer Research* 61(9): 3689–97.

20. J. Landreneau et al. (2015), "Immunological Mechanisms of Low and Ultra-Low Dose Cancer Chemotherapy," *Cancer Microenvironment* 8(2): 57–64.

21. V. R. Rozados et al. (2004), "Metronomic Therapy with Cyclophosphamide Induces Rat Lymphoma and Sarcoma Regression, and Is Devoid of Toxicity," *Annals of Oncology* 15(10): 1543–50.

22. P. Malik et al. (2014), "Metronomics as Maintenance Treatment in Oncology: Time for Chemo-Switch," *Frontiers in Oncology* 4: 1–7.

23. R. S. Kerbel and B. A. Kamen (2004), "The Anti-Angiogenic Basis of Metronomic Chemotherapy," *Nature Reviews Cancer* 4(6): 423–36.

24. M. Colleoni et al. (2002), "Low-Dose Oral Methotrexate and Cyclophosphamide in Metastatic Breast Cancer: Antitumor Activity and Correlation with Vascular Endothelial Growth Factor Levels," *Annals of Oncology* 13(1): 73–80.

25. F. Ghiringhell et al. (2007), "Metronomic Cyclophosphamide Regimen Selectively Depletes CD4+CD25+ Regulatory T Cells and Restores T and NK Effector Functions in End Stage Cancer Patients," *Cancer Immunology, Immunotherapy* 56(5): 641–48.

26. O. Laura et al. (2006), "Prolonged Clinical Benefit with Metronomic Chemotherapy in Patients with Metastatic Breast Cancer," *Anti-Cancer Drugs* 17(8): 961–67.

27. S. Dellapasqua et al. (2008), "Metronomic Cyclophosphamide and Capecitabine Combined with Bevacizumab in Advanced Breast Cancer," *Journal of Clinical Oncology* 26(30): 4899–905.

28. J. Chura et al. (2007), "Bevacizumab Plus Cyclophosphamide in Heavily Pretreated Patients with Recurrent Ovarian Cancer," *Gynecologic Oncology* 107(2): 326–30.

29. L. Simkens (2015), "Maintenance Treatment with Capecitabine and Bevacizumab in Metastatic Colorectal Cancer (CAIRO3): A Phase 3 Randomised Controlled Trial of the Dutch Colorectal Cancer Group," *Lancet* 385(9980): 1843–52.

30. S. Dellapasqua et al. (2008), "Metronomic Cyclophosphamide and Capecitabine Combined with Bevacizumab in Advanced Breast Cancer," *Journal of Clinical Oncology* 26(30): 4899–905.

31. S. Kummar (2011), "Multihistology, Target-Driven Pilot Trial of Oral Topotecan as an Inhibitor of Hypoxia-Inducible Factor-1α in Advanced Solid," *Cancer Research* 17(15): 5123–31.

4. EAST MEETS WEST

1. U. Jaffer et al. (2010), "Cytokines in the Systemic Inflammatory Response Syndrome: A Review," *HSR Proceedings in Intensive Care & Cardiovascular Anesthesia* 2(3): 161–75.

2. J. Morley et al. (2006), "Cachexia: Pathophysiology and Clinical Relevance 1,2," *American Journal of Clinical Nutrition* 83(4): 735–43.

3. A. Nicolinia et al. (2013), "Malnutrition, Anorexia, and Cachexia in Cancer Patients: A Mini-Review on Pathogenesis and Treatment," *Biomedicine & Pharmacotherapy* 67(8): 807–17.

4. R. Nemade et al. (2007), "Classic Symptoms of Major Depression," MentalHealth.net.

5. J. Giese-Davis et al. (2011), "Decrease in Depression Symptoms Is Associated with Longer Survival in Patients with Metastatic Breast Cancer: A Secondary Analysis," *Journal of Clinical Oncology* 29(4): 413–20.

6. R. Cheng (2014), "Traditional Chinese Medicine Basics."

7. T. Lahans (2007), *Integrating Conventional and Chinese Medicine in Cancer Care: A Clinical Guide* (Philadelphia: Churchill Livingstone Elsevier).

8. J. P. Briggs (2014), "The Evidence Base for Integrative Approaches to Cancer Care," U.S. Department of Health and Human Services, National Institutes of Health, National Center for Complementary and Integrative Health (NCCIH).

9. K. Wong et al. (2004), "Immunomodulatory Effects of *yun zhi* and *danshen* Capsules in Health Subjects—A Randomized, Double-Blind, Placebo-Controlled, Crossover Study," *International Immunopharmacology* 4(2): 201–11.

10. T. S. Lee (2017), "Principles of Naturopathic Medicine," Naturo.doc.

11. T. Ming-Ju et al. (2014), "Tumor Microenvironment: A New Treatment Target for Cancer," *ISRN Biochemistry* 2014, Article ID 351959.

12. M. Nowacki et al. (1996), "Inflammation and Metastases," *Medical Hypotheses* 47(3): 193–96.

13. H. Adair and P. Montani (2010), *Angiogenesis* (San Rafael, CA: Morgan & Claypool Life Sciences).

14. E. Hayden (2009), "Cutting Off Cancer's Supply Lines," *Nature* 458(7239): 686–87.

15. T. Byers et al. (2001), "American Cancer Society Guidelines on Nutrition and Physical Activity for Cancer Prevention: Reducing the Risk of Cancer with Healthy Food Choices and Physical Activity," *A Cancer Journal for Clinicians* 52(2): 92–119.

16. T. Byers et al. (2001), "American Cancer Society Guidelines on Nutrition and Physical Activity for Cancer Prevention: Reducing the Risk of Cancer with Healthy Food Choices and Physical Activity," *A Cancer Journal for Clinicians* 52(2): 92–119.

17. American Institute for Cancer Research (2017), "Recommendations for Cancer Prevention."

18. B. G. Allen et al. (2014), "Ketogenic Diets as an Adjuvant Cancer Therapy: History and Potential Mechanism," *Redox Biology* 2 (2014): 963–70.

19. M. Schmidt et al. (2011), "Effects of a Ketogenic Diet on the Quality of Life in 16 Patients with Advanced Cancer: A Pilot Trial," *Nutrition & Metabolism* 8(1): 54.

20. G. Zuccoli et al. (2010), "Metabolic Management of Glioblastoma Multiforme Using Standard Therapy Together with a Restricted Ketogenic Diet: Case Report," *Nutrition & Metabolism* 7(1): 33.

21. S. Zhou et al. (2007), "Frequency and Phenotypic Implications of Mitochondrial DNA Mutations in Human Squamous Cell Cancers of the Head and Neck," *Proceedings of the National Academy of Sciences of the United States of America* 104(18): 7540–45.

22. S. Patel and A. Goyal (2011), "Recent Developments in Mushroom as Anti-Cancer Therapeutics: A Review," *3 Biotech* 2(1): 1–15.

23. D. C. Brown and J. Reetz (2012), "Single Agent Polysaccharopeptide Delays Metastases and Improves Survival in Naturally Occurring Hemangiosarcoma," *Evidence-Based Complementary and Alternative Medicine* 2012(5): 1–8.

24. M. R. C. G. Novaes et al. (2011), "The Effects of Dietary Supplementation with Agaricales Mushrooms and Other Medicinal Fungi on Breast Cancer: Evidence-Based Medicine," *Clinics* 66(12): 2133–39.

25. Z. Yin et al. (2010), "Effects of Active Hexose Correlated Compound on Frequency of CD4+ and CD8+ T Cells Producing Interferon-γ and/or Tumor Necrosis Factor-α in Healthy Adults," *Human Immunology* 71(12): 1187–90.

26. R. A. Sharma et al. (2007), "Pharrmacokinetics and Pharmacodynamics of Curcumin," in *The Molecular Targets and Therapeutic Uses of Curcumin in Health and Disease*, edited by B. B. Aggarwal et al. (New York: Springer).

27. J. Asha et al. (2007), "Mechanism of the Anti-Inflammatory Effect of Curcumin: PPAR-γ Activation," *PPAR Research* 2007(1): 1–5.

28. R. M. Srivastavaa et al. (2011), "Immunomodulatory and Therapeutic Activity of Curcumin," *International Immunopharmacology* 11(3): 331–41.

29. N. Fleshner and A. R. Zlotta (2007), "Prostate Cancer Prevention," *Cancer* 110: 1889–99.

30. N. Tang et al. (2009), "Green Tea, Black Tea Consumption and Risk of Lung Cancer: A Meta-Analysis," *Lung Cancer* 65(3): 274–83.

31. M. J. Li et al. (2014), "Green Tea Compounds in Breast Cancer Prevention and Treatment," *World Journal of Clinical Oncology* 5(3): 520–28.

32. K. Tallmadge (2013), "Understanding the Power of Omega-3s" (Op-Ed). Livescience.com.

33. P. J. Skerrett (2014), "Selenium, Vitamin E Supplements Increase Prostate Cancer Risk," Harvard Health Blog.

34. C. M. Doskey et al. (2016), "Tumor Cells Have Decreased Ability to Metabolize H2O2: Implications for Pharmacological Ascorbate in Cancer Therapy," *Redox Biology* 10(2): 274–84.

35. C. M. Doskey et al. (2016), "Tumor Cells Have Decreased Ability to Metabolize H2O2: Implications for Pharmacological Ascorbate in Cancer Therapy," *Redox Biology* 10(2): 274–84.

36. M. Levine (2006), "Prolonged Survival Linked to Intravenous Vitamin C Seen in Three Cancer Patients," *Canadian Medical Association Journal* 174: 937–42.

37. Q. Chen et al. (2008), "Pharmacologic Doses of Ascorbate Act as a Pro-Oxidant and Decrease Growth of Aggressive Tumor Xenografts in Mice." *Proceedings National Academy of Sciences of the United States of America* 105(32): 11105–109.

38. V. I. Lushchak (2012), "Glutathione Homeostasis and Functions: Potential Targets for Medical Interventions," *Journal of Amino Acids* 2012(5): 1–26.

39. L. N. Alschuler and K. A. Gazella (2010), *Definitive Guide to Cancer: An Integrative Approach to Prevention, Treatment, and Healing* (Las Vegas, NV: Celestial Arts).

40. W. Dröge et al. (1996), "Role of Cysteine and Glutathione in HIV Infection and Cancer Cachexia: Therapeutic Intervention with N-Acetylcysteine," *Advances in Pharmacology* 38(1996): 581–600.

41. B. D. Lawenda et al. (2008), "Should Supplemental Antioxidant Administration Be Avoided during Chemotherapy and Radiation Therapy?" *Journal of the National Cancer Institute* 100(11): 773–83.

42. K. Gaurav et al. (2012), "Glutamine: A Novel Approach to Chemotherapy-Induced Toxicity," *Indian Journal of Medical and Paediatric Oncology* 33(1): 13–20.

43. E. Bach (1987), *Collected Writings of Edward Bach*, edited by Julian Barnard (Bath, UK: Ashgrove). Excellent reading, philosophy, and practical information on the remedies.

44. P. Lissoni et al. (2003), "Five Years Survival in Metastatic Non-Small Cell Lung Cancer Patients Treated with Chemotherapy Alone or Chemotherapy and Melatonin: A Randomized Trial," *Journal of Pineal Research* 35(1): 12–15.

45. N. Morgan et al. (2007), "Implementing an Expressive Writing Study in a Cancer Clinic," *The Oncologist* 13(2): 196–204.

5. INTEGRATIVE TREATMENT PLANS
IN ACTION

1. R. S. Kerbel (2014), "Development and Evolution of the Concept of Metronomic Chemotherapy: A Personal Perspective," in *Metronomic Chemotherapy*, edited by G. Bocci and G. Francia (Berlin, Heidelberg: Springer).

2. D. Mauri et al. (2010), "Overall Survival Benefit for Weekly vs. Three-Weekly Taxanes Regimens in Advanced Breast Cancer: A Meta-Analysis." *Cancer Treatment Reviews* 36(1): 69–74.

3. S. Pignata et al. (2013), "A Randomized Multicenter Phase III Study Comparing Weekly versus Every 3 Weeks Carboplatin (C) Plus Paclitaxel (P) in Patients with Advanced Ovarian Cancer (AOC): Multicenter Italian Trials in Ovarian Cancer (MITO-7)—European Network of Gynaecological Oncological Trial Groups (ENGOT-ov-10) and Gynecologic Cancer Intergroup (GCIG) Trial," ASCO 2013, Abstract LBA5501,

4. N. Chen (2008), "Prolonged Metronomic Chemotherapy in Advanced Non-Small-Cell Lung Cancer Is Associated with Excellent Long-Term Survival," *Clinical Lung Cancer* 9(5): 290.

5. D. Kang et al. (2010), "Significant Impairment in Immune Recovery Following Cancer Treatment," *Nursing Research* 58(2): 105–14.

6. SEER 18 2007–2013, All Races, Females by SEER Summary Stage 2000.

7. T. Creagan et al. (1979), "Failure of High-Dose Vitamin C (Ascorbic Acid) Therapy to Benefit Patients with Advanced Cancer: A Controlled Trial," *New England Journal of Medicine* 301(13): 687–90.

8. Q. Chen et al. (2017), "Pharmacologic Ascorbic Acid Concentrations Selectively Kill Cancer Cells: Action as a Pro-Drug to Deliver Hydrogen Peroxide to Tissues," *Proceedings of the National Academy of Science of the United States of America* 102(38): 13604–9.

9. L. Cimmino et al. (2017), "Restoration of TET2 Function Blocks Aberrant Self-Renewal and Leukemia Progression," *Cell* 170(6): 939–55.

10. H. Kang et al. (2013), "The Critical Role of Catalase in Prooxidant and Antioxidant Function of p53," *Cell Death and Differentiation* 20(1): 117–29.

6. MOVING FORWARD WITH INTEGRATIVE CANCER TREATMENT

1. C. Tokheima et al. (2016), "Evaluating the Evaluation of Cancer Driver Genes," *Proceedings of the National Academy of Sciences of the United States* 113: 14330–35.

2. R. Rosell et al. (2012), "Erlotinib versus Standard Chemotherapy as First-Line Treatment for European Patients with Advanced EGFR Mutation-Positive Non-Small-Cell Lung Cancer (EURTAC): A Multicentre, Open-Label, Randomised Phase 3 Trial," *Lancet* 13(3): 239–46.

3. S. Herbst et al. (2005), "A Phase III Trial of Erlotinib Hydrochloride (OSI-774) Combined with Carboplatin and Paclitaxel Chemotherapy in Advanced Non-Small-Cell Lung Cancer," *Journal of Clinical Oncology* 23(25): 5892–99.

4. E. Pasquier et al. (2010), "Metronomic Chemotherapy: New Rationale for New Directions," *Nature Reviews Clinical Oncology* 7(8): 455–65.

5. J. Galon (2006), "Type, Density, and Location of Immune Cells within Human Colorectal Tumors Predict Clinical Outcome," *Science* 313(5795): 1960–64.

6. D. Pardoll (2012), "The Blockade of Immune Checkpoints in Cancer Immunotherapy," *Nature Reviews Cancer* 12(4): 252.

7. S. Hodi et al. (2010), "Improved Survival with Ipilimumab in Patients with Metastatic Melanoma," *The New England Journal of Medicine* 363(8): 711–23.

8. J. Brahmer et al. (2015), "Nivolumab versus Docetaxel in Advanced Squamous-Cell Non–Small-Cell Lung Cancer," *New England Journal of Medicine* 373(2): 123–35.

9. S. Patel and R. Kurzrock (2015), "PD-L1 Expression as a Predictive Biomarker in Cancer Immunotherapy," *Molecular Cancer Therapeutics* 14(4): 847–56.

10. S. Kalathil et al. (2013), "Higher Frequencies of GARP+CTLA-4+Foxp3+ T Regulatory Cells and Myeloid-Derived Suppressor Cells in Hepatocellular Carcinoma Patients Are Associated with Impaired T-Cell Functionality," *Cancer Research* 73(8): 2435–44.

11. National Cancer Institute (2017), "CAR T Cells: Engineering Patients' Immune Cells to Treat Their Cancers."

Q & A

1. National Institutes of Health.
2. National Institutes of Health.

BIBLIOGRAPHY

CHAPTER 1:
FROM MUSTARD GAS TO MODERN MEDICINE

Bonadonna, G., Valagussa, P., Moliterni, A., Zambetti, M., and Brambilla, C. (1995). "Adjuvant Cyclophosphamide, Methotrexate, and Fluorouracil in Node-Positive Breast Cancer: The Results of 20 Years of Follow-Up." *New England Journal of Medicine* 332(14): 901–6.

Cao, Y., and Langer, R. (2008). "A Review of Judah Folkman's Remarkable Achievements in Biomedicine." *Proceedings of the National Academy of Sciences of the United States of America* 105(36): 13203–5.

Carter, J. S. (2014). "Mitosis." http://biology.clc.uc.edu/courses/bio104/mitosis.htm.

Christa, P. (2011). "The Birth of Chemotherapy at Yale." Bicentennial Lecture Series: Surgery Grand Round. *Yale Journal of Biology and Medicine* 84(2): 169–72.

DeVita, V., and Chu, E. (2008). "A History of Cancer Chemotherapy." *Cancer Rearch* 68(21): 8643–53.

Fisher, B., Costantino, J., Redmond, C., Fisher, E., Margolese, R., Dimitrov, N., Wolmark, N., Wickerham, D., Deutsch, M., Ore, L., Mamounas, E., Poller, W., and Kavanah, M. (1993). "Lumpectomy Compared with Lumpectomy and Radiation Therapy for the Treatment of Intraductal Breast Cancer." *New England Journal of Medicine* 328(22): 1581–86. doi:10.1056/NEJM199306033282201.

Freireich, E. (2002). "Special Article: Min Chiu Li—A Perspective in Cancer Therapy." *Clinical Cancer Research* 8(9): 2764–65.

Heron, M., Hoyert, D., Murphy, S., Xu, J., Kochanek, K., and Tejada-Vera, B. (2006). "Deaths: Final Data for 2006." *National Vital Statistics Reports* 57(14): 1–134.

Li, M. C., Hertz, R., and Spencer, D. B. (1956). "Effect of Methotrexate Therapy upon Choriocarcinoma and Chorioadenoma." *Proceedings of the Society for Experimental Biology and Medicine* 93(2): 361–66. PMID 13379512. doi:10.3181/00379727-93-22757.

Nussey, S., and Whitehead, S. (2001). *Endocrinology: An Integrated Approach.* Oxford, UK: BIOS Scientific Publishers Limited.

Weisse, A. B. (1991). *Medical Odysseys: The Different and Sometimes Unexpected Pathways to Twentieth-Century Medical Discoveries.* New Brunswick, NJ: Rutgers University Press.

CHAPTER 2:
IN DEFENSE OF OUR HEALTH

Arap, M., Lahdenranta, J., Mintz, P., Hajitou, A., Sarkis, A., Arap, W., and Pasqualini, R. (2004). "Cell Surface Expression of the Stress Response Chaperone GRP78 Enables Tumor Targeting by Circulating Ligands." *Cancer Cell* 6(3): 275–84. https://doi.org/10.1016/j.ccr. 2004.08.018.

Bhatia, A., and Kumar, Y. (2011). "Cancer-Immune Equilibrium: Questions Unanswered." *Cancer Microenvironment* 4(2): 209–17. http://doi.org/10.1007/s12307-011-0065-8.

Chandan, V., Kaewkangsadan, V., Eremin, L., Cowley, G., Ilyas, M., El-Sheemy, M., and Eremin, O. (2015). "Natural Killer (NK) Cell Profiles in Blood and Tumour in Women with Large and Locally Advanced Breast Cancer (LLABC) and Their Contribution to a Pathological Complete Response (PCR) in the Tumour Following Neoadjuvant Chemotherapy (NAC): Differential Restoration of Blood Profiles by NAC and Surgery." *Journal of Translational Medicine* 13(1): 1–21.

Duck-Hee, K., Weaver, M., Na-Jin, P., Smith, B., McArdle, T., and Carpenter. J. (2009). "Significant Impairment in Immune Recovery Following Cancer Treatment." *Nursing Research* 58(2): 105–14. doi:10.1097/NNR.0b013e31818fceed.

Dunn, G., Bruce, A., Ikeda, H., Old, L., and Schreiber, R. (2002). "Cancer Immunoediting: From Immunosurveillance to Tumor Escape." *Nature Immunology* 3(11): 991–98. doi:10.1038/ni1102-991.

Fu, D., Geschwind, J. F., Karthikeyan, S., Miller, E., Kunjithapatham, R., Wang, Z., and Ganapathy-Kanniappan, S. (2015). "Metabolic Perturbation Sensitizes Human Breast Cancer to NK Cell-Mediated Cytotoxicity by Increasing the Expression of MHC Class I Chain-Related A/B." *Oncoimmunology* 4(3): 1–10. doi:10.4161/2162402X.2014.991228.

Hulsewé, K. W., van Acker, B. A., von Meyenfeldt, M. F., and Soeters, P. B. (1999). "Nutritional Depletion and Dietary Manipulation: Effects on the Immune Response." *World Journal of Surgery* 23(6): 536–44. https://doi.org/10.1007/PL00012344.

Imai, K., Satoru, M., Satoshi, M., Kenji, S., and Kei, N. (2000). "Natural Cytotoxic Activity of Peripheral-Blood Lymphocytes and Cancer Incidence: An 11-Year Follow-Up Study of a General Population." *Lancet* 356(9244): 1795–99. doi:10.1016/S0140-6736(00)03231-1.

Jobin, G., Rodriguez-Suarez, R., and Betito, K. (2017). "Association between Natural Killer Cell Activity and Colorectal Cancer in High-Risk Subjects Undergoing Colonoscopy." *Gastroenterology* 153(4): 980–87. https://doi.org/10.1053/j.gastro.2017.06.009.

Lanier, L. L. (2015). "NKG2D Receptor and Its Ligands in Host Defense." *Cancer Immunology Research* 3(6): 575–82. http://doi.org/10.1158/2326-6066.CIR-15-0098.

Pulendran, B., and Ahmed, R. (2006). "Review Translating Innate Immunity into Immunological Memory: Implications for Vaccine Development." *Cell* 124(4): 849–63. https://doi.org/ 10.1016/j.cell.2006.02.019..

Ryungsa, K., Kawai, A., Wakisaka, M., Garaku, H., Yasuda, N., Ohtani,S., Ito, M., and Arihiro, K. (2016). "A Role for Peripheral Natural Killer (NK) Cell Activity in the Response to Neoadjuvant Chemotherapy in Patients with Breast Cancer." *Journal of Clinical Oncology* 34(15): e12073.

Vesely, M. D., Kershaw, M. H., Schreiber, R. D., and Smyth, M. J. (2010). "Natural Innate and Adaptive Immunity to Cancer." *Annual Review of Immunology* 29: 235–71. PMID: 21219185.

CHAPTER 3:
LESS IS MORE

Amy, K. (2016). "Tumor-Induced MDSC Act via Remote Control to Inhibit L-Selectin-Dependent Adaptive 2 Immunity in Lymph Nodes." *eLife* 5: e17375. Published online December 8, 2016. doi:10.7554/eLife.17375.

Bertolini, F. (2003). "Maximum Tolerable Dose and Low-Dose Metronomic Chemotherapy Have Opposite Effects on the Mobilization and Viability of Circulating Endothelial Progenitor Cells." *Cancer Research* 63(15): 4342–46.

Browder, T., Butterfield, E., Kräling, M., Shi, B., Marshall, B., O'Reilly, M. S., and Folkman, J. (2000). "Antiangiogenic Scheduling of Chemotherapy Improves Efficacy against Experimental Drug-Resistant Cancer." *Cancer Research* 60(7): 1878–86.

Chan, T. S., Hsu, C. C., Pai, V. C., Liao, W. Y., Huang, S. S., Tan, K. T., and Tsai, K-C. (2016). "Metronomic Chemotherapy Prevents Therapy-Induced Stromal Activation and Induction of Tumor-Initiating Cells." *Journal of Experimental Medicine* 213(13): 2967–88. doi:10.1084/jem.20151665.

Chung, A., et al. (2012). "Differential Drug Class-Specific Metastatic Effects Following Treatment with a Panel of Angiogenesis Inhibitors." *The Journal of Pathology* 227(4): 404–16.

Chura, J., et al. (2007). "Bevacizumab Plus Cyclophosphamide in Heavily Pretreated Patients with Recurrent Ovarian Cancer." *Gynecologic Oncology* 107(2): 326–30.

Citron, M., Berry, D., Cirrincione, C., Hudis, C., Winer, E., Gradishar, W., Davidson, N., Martino, S., Livingston, R., Ingle, J., Perez, R., Carpenter, J., Hurd, D., Holland, J., Smith, B., Sartor, C., Leung, E., Abrams, J., Schilsky, R., Muss, H., and Norton, L. (2003). "Randomized Trial of Dose-Dense versus Conventionally Scheduled and Sequential versus Concurrent Combination Chemotherapy as Postoperative Adjuvant Treatment of Node-Positive Primary Breast Cancer: First Report of Intergroup Trial C9741/Cancer and Leukemia Group B Trial 9741." *Journal of Clinical Oncology* 21(8): 1431–39.

Colleoni, M., et al. (2002). "Low-Dose Oral Methotrexate and Cyclophosphamide in Metastatic Breast Cancer: Antitumor Activity and Correlation with Vascular Endothelial Growth Factor Levels." *Annals of Oncology* 13(1): 73–80.

Dellapasqua, S. J., et al. (2008). "Metronomic Cyclophosphamide and Capecitabine Combined with Bevacizumab in Advanced Breast Cancer." *Clinical Oncology* 26(30): 4899–905.

Emens, L. A., Asquith, J. M., Leatherman, J. M., Kobrin, B. J., Petrik, S., Laiko, M., . . . Jaffee, E. M. (2009). "Timed Sequential Treatment with Cyclophosphamide, Doxorubicin, and an Allogeneic Granulocyte-Macrophage Colony-Stimulating Factor-Secreting Breast Tumor Vaccine: A Chemotherapy Dose-Ranging Factorial Study of Safety and Immune Activation." *Journal of Clinical Oncology* 27(35): 5911–18. doi:10.1200/JCO.2009.23.3494.

Gammon, K. (2012). "Mathematical Modelling: Forecasting Cancer." *Nature* 491(7425): S66–S67. doi:10.1038/491S66a491S66a.

Ghiringhell, F., et al. (2007). "Metronomic Cyclophosphamide Regimen Selectively Depletes CD4+CD25+ Regulatory T Cells and Restores T and NK Effector Functions in End Stage Cancer Patients." *Cancer Immunology, Immunotherapy* 56(5): 641–48.

Kerbel, R. S., and Kamen, B. A. (2004). "The Anti-Angiogenic Basis of Metronomic Chemotherapy." *Nature Reviews Cancer* 4(6): 423–36. doi:10.1038/nrc1369.

Kerbel, R., Klement, G., Pritchard, K., and Kamen, B. (2002). "Continuous Low-Dose Anti-Angiogenic/Metronomic Chemotherapy: From the Research Laboratory into the Oncology Clinic." *Annals of Oncology* 13(1): 12–15.

Klement, G., Huang, P., Mayer, B., Green, K., Man, S., Bohlen. P., Hicklin, D., and Kerbel, S. (2002). "Differences in Therapeutic Indexes of Combination Metronomic Chemotherapy and an Anti-VEGFR-2 Antibody in Multidrug-Resistant Human Breast Cancer Xenografts." *Clinical Cancer Research* 8(1): 221–32.

Kummar, S. (2011). "Multihistology: Target-Driven Pilot Trial of Oral Topotecan as an Inhibitor of Hypoxia-Inducible Factor-1α in Advanced Solid." *Cancer Research* 17(15): 5123–31.

Landreneau, J., et al. (2015). "Immunological Mechanisms of Low and Ultra-Low Dose Cancer Chemotherapy." *Cancer Microenvironment* 8(2): 57–64.

Licun, Wu. (2011). "Tumor Cell Repopulation between Cycles of Chemotherapy Is Inhibited by Regulatory T-Cell Depletion in a Murine Mesothelioma Model." *Journal of Thoracic Oncology* 6(9): 1578–86.

Laura, O., et al. (2006). "Prolonged Clinical Benefit with Metronomic Chemotherapy in Patients with Metastatic Breast Cancer." *Anti-Cancer Drugs* 17(8): 961–67.

Machiels, J. P. H., Todd Reilly, R., Emens, L. A., Ercolini, A. M., Lei, R. Y., Weintraub, D., and Jaffee, E. M. (2001). "Cyclophosphamide, Doxorubicin, and Paclitaxel Enhance the Antitumor Immune Response of Granulocyte/Macrophage-Colony Stimulating Factor-Secreting Whole-Cell Vaccines in HER-2/Neu Tolerized Mice." *Cancer Research* 61(9): 3689–97.

Malik, P., Raina, V., and Nicolas, A. (2014). "Metronomics as Maintenance Treatment in Oncology: Time for Chemo-Switch." *Frontiers in Oncology* 4: 1–7.

Michele, L. (2010). "Conditional Regulatory T-Cell Depletion Releases Adaptive Immunity Preventing Carcinogenesis and Suppressing Established Tumor Growth." *Cancer Research* 70(20): 7800–09.

Rozados, V. R., et al. (2004). "Metronomic Therapy with Cyclophosphamide Induces Rat Lymphoma and Sarcoma Regression, and Is Devoid of Toxicity." *Annals of Oncology* 15(10): 1543–50.

Sennino, B., Raatschen, J., Wendland, F., Fu, Y., You, K., Shames, M., McDonald, M., and Brasch, C. (2009). "Correlative Dynamic Contrast MRI and Microscopic Assessments of Tumor Vascularity in RIP-Tag2 Transgenic Mice." *Magnetic Resonance in Medicine* 62(3): 616–25.

Simkens, L. (2015). "Maintenance Treatment with Capecitabine and Bevacizumab in Metastatic Colorectal Cancer (CAIRO3): A Phase 3 Randomised Controlled Trial of the Dutch Colorectal Cancer Group." *Lancet* 385(9980): 1843–52.

Simon, R., and Norton, L. (2006). "The Norton–Simon Hypothesis: Designing More Effective and Less Toxic Chemotherapeutic Regimens." *Nature Clinical Practice Oncology* 3(8): 406–07.

Skipper, H., Schabel, F., and Wilcox, W. (1964). "Experimental Evaluation of Potential Anticancer Agents. XIII: On the Criteria and Kinetics Associated with 'Curability' of Experimental Leukemia." *Cancer Chemotherapy Reports* 35: 1–111.

Vedran, R., et al. (2010). "Cyclophosphamide Resets Dendritic Cell Homeostasis and Enhances Antitumor Immunity through Effects That Extend Beyond Regulatory T Cell Elimination." *Cancer Immunology, Immunotherapy* 59(1): 137–48.

Vicari, P. (2009). "Paclitaxel Reduces Regulatory T Cell Numbers and Inhibitory Function and Enhances the Anti-Tumor Effects of the TLR9 Agonist PF-3512676 in the Mouse." *Cancer Immunology, Immunotherapy* 58(4): 615–28. doi:10.1007/s00262-008-0586-2. Epub September 19, 2008.

Xavier, V., et al. (2007). "Deficient CD4+CD25high T Regulatory Cell Function in Patients with Active Systemic Lupus Erythematosus." *Journal of Immunology* 178(4): 2579–88.

CHAPTER 4:
EAST MEETS WEST

Adair, H., and Montani, P. (2010). *Angiogenesis*. San Rafael, CA: Morgan & Claypool Life Sciences. Available from https://www.ncbi.nlm.nih.gov/books/NBK53242/.

Allen, B. G., Bhatia, S. K., Anderson, C. M., Eichenberger-Gilmore, J. M., Sibenaller, Z. A., Mapuskar, K. A., Schoenfeld, J. D., Buatti, J. M., Spitz, D. R., and Fath, M. A. (2014). "Ketogenic Diets as an Adjuvant Cancer Therapy: History and Potential Mechanism." *Redox Biology* 2 (2014): 963–70. http://www.sciencedirect.com/science/article/pii/S2213231714000925.

Alschuler, L. N., and Gazella, K. A. (2010). *Definitive Guide to Cancer, 3rd Edition: An Integrative Approach to Prevention, Treatment, and Healing.* Las Vegas, NV: Celestial Arts.

American Institute for Cancer Research. (2017). "Recommendations for Cancer Prevention." http://www.aicr.org/reduce-your-cancer-risk/recommendations-for-cancer-prevention/recommendations_04_plant_based.html.

Asha, J., Rongqian, W., and Ping, W. (2009). "Mechanism of the Anti-Inflammatory Effect of Curcumin: PPAR-γ Activation." *PPAR Research* 2007(1): 1–5. https://doi.org/10.1007/s11888-009-0002-0.

Bach, E. (1987). *Collected Writings of Edward Bach,* edited by Julian Barnard. Bath, UK: Ashgrove.

Briggs, J. P. (2014). "The Evidence Base for Integrative Approaches to Cancer Care." U.S. Department of Health and Human Services, National Institutes of Health, National Center for Complementary and Integrative Health (NCCIH). November 20, 2014. https://nccih.nih.gov/research/blog/cancer-integrative-care.

Brown, D. C., and Reetz, J. (2012). "Single Agent Polysaccharopeptide Delays Metastases and Improves Survival in Naturally Occurring Hemangiosarcoma." *Evidence-Based Complementary and Alternative Medicine* 2012(5): 1–8. doi:10.1155/2012/384301.

Byers, T., Nestle, M., McTiernan, A., Doyle, C., Currie-Williams, A., Gansler, T., and Thun, M. (2001). "American Cancer Society Guidelines on Nutrition and Physical Activity for Cancer Prevention: Reducing the Risk of Cancer with Healthy Food. Choices and Physical Activity." *A Cancer Journal for Clinicians* 52(2): 92–119.

Chen, Q., Graham, M., Sun, A., Chaya, P., Kirk, K., Krishna, M., Khosh, D., Drisko, J. and Levine, M. (2008). "Pharmacologic Doses of Ascorbate Act as a Pro-Oxidant and Decrease Growth of Aggressive Tumor Xenografts in Mice." *Proceedings National Academy of Sciences of the United States of America* 105(32): 11105–09.

Cheng, R. (2014). "Traditional Chinese Medicine Basics." http://www.tcmbasics.com/etiology.htm.

Doskey, C. M., Buranasudja, V., Wagner, B. A., Wilkes, J. G., Du, J., Cullen, J. J., and Buettner, G. R. "Tumor Cells Have Decreased Ability to Metabolize H2O2: Implications for Pharmacological Ascorbate in Cancer Therapy." *Redox Biology* 10(2): 274–84. doi:10.1016/j.redox.2016.10.010.

Dröge, W., Gross, A., Hack, V., Kinsche, R., Schykowski, M., Bockstett, M., Mihm, S.,and Galte, D. (1996). "Role of Cysteine and Glutathione in HIV Infection and Cancer Cachexia: Therapeutic Intervention with N-Acetylcysteine." *Advances in Pharmacology* 38(1996): 581–600.

Fleshner, N., and Zlotta, A. R. (2007). "Prostate Cancer Prevention." *Cancer* 110: 1889–99. doi:10.1002/cncr.23009.

Gaurav, K., Goel, R. K., Shukla, M., and Pandey, M. (2012). "Glutamine: A Novel Approach to Chemotherapy-Induced Toxicity." *Indian Journal of Medical and Paediatric Oncology* 33(1): 13–20.

Giese-Davis, J., Collie, K., Rancourt, K., Neri, E., Kraemer, H., and Spiegel, D. (2011). "Decrease in Depression Symptoms Is Associated with Longer Survival in Patients with Metastatic Breast Cancer: A Secondary Analysis." *Journal of Clinical Oncology* 29(4): 413–20. doi:10.1200/JCO.2010.28.4455.

Hayden, E. (2009). "Cutting Off Cancer's Supply Lines." *Nature* 458(7239): 686–87. PMID 19360048. doi:10.1038/458686b.

Jaffer, U., Wade, R. G., and Gourlay, T. (2010). "Cytokines in the Systemic Inflammatory Response Syndrome: A Review." *HSR Proceedings in Intensive Care & Cardiovascular Anesthesia* 2(3): 161–75.

Wang, J.,Wang, X., Jiang, S., Lin, P., Zhang, J., Lu, Y., Wang, Q., Xiong, Z., Wu, Y., Ren, J., and Yang, H. (2008). "Cytotoxicity of Fig Fruit Latex against Human Cancer Cells." *Food and Chemical Toxicology* 46(3): 1025–33.

Lahans, T. (2007). *Integrating Conventional and Chinese Medicine in Cancer Care: A Clinical Guide.* Philadelphia: Churchill Livingstone Elsevier.

Lawenda, B. D., Kelly, K. M., Ladas, E. J., Sagar, S. M., Vickers, A., and Blumberg, J. B. (2008). "Should Supplemental Antioxidant Administration Be Avoided during Chemotherapy and Radiation Therapy?" *Journal of the National Cancer Institute* 100(11): 773–83. https://doi.org/10.1093/jnci/djn148.

Lee, T. S. (2017). "Principles of Naturopathic Medicine." Naturo.doc. http://www.naturodoc.com/cardinal/naturopathy/nat_principles.htm.

Levine, M. (2006). "Prolonged Survival Linked to Intravenous Vitamin C Seen in Three Cancer Patients." *Canadian Medical Association Journal* 174: 937–42.

Li, M. J., Yin, Y. C., Wang, J., and Jiang, Y. F. (2014). "Green Tea Compounds in Breast Cancer Prevention and Treatment." *World Journal of Clinical Oncology* 5(3): 520–28.

Lissoni, P., Chilelli, M., Villa, S., Cerizza, L., and Tancini, G. (2003). "Five Years Survival in Metastatic Non-Small Cell Lung Cancer Patients Treated with Chemotherapy Alone or Chemotherapy and Melatonin: A Randomized Trial." *Journal of Pineal Research* 35(1): 12–15.

Lushchak, V. I. (2012). "Glutathione Homeostasis and Functions: Potential Targets for Medical Interventions." *Journal of Amino Acids* 2012(5): 1–26. http://dx.doi.org/10.1155/2012/736837.

Milner, J. A. (1996). "Garlic: Its Anticarcinogenic and Antitumorigenic Properties." *Nutrition Reviews* 54(11): S82–S86.

Ming-Ju, T., Wei-An, C., Ming-Shyan, H., and Po-Lin, K. (2014). "Tumor Microenvironment: A New Treatment Target for Cancer." *Biochemistry* 2014, Article ID 351959. doi:10.1155/2014/351959.

Morgan, N., Graves, K., Poggi, E., and Cheson, B. (2007). "Implementing an Expressive Writing Study in a Cancer Clinic." *The Oncologist* 13(2): 196–204.

Morley, J., Thomas, D., and Wilson, M. (2006). "Cachexia: Pathophysiology and Clinical Relevance1,2." *American Journal of Clinical Nutrition* 83(4): 735–43.

Nemade, R., Staats, N., and Dombeck, M. (2007). "Classic Symptoms of Major Depression." MentalHealth.net. https://www.mentalhelp.net/articles/psychology-of-depression-psycho dynamic-theories/.

Nicolinia, A., Ferraria, P., Chiara, M., Milena, M., Stefania, F., Ottavio, P., and Angelo, G. (2013). "Malnutrition, Anorexia and Cachexia in Cancer Patients: A Mini-Review on Pathogenesis and Treatment." *Biomedicine & Pharmacotherapy* 67(8): 807–17.

Novaes, M. R. C. G., Valadares, F., Reis, M. C., Gonçalves, D. R., Menezes, M. C. (2011). "The Effects of Dietary Supplementation with Agaricales Mushrooms and Other Medicinal Fungi on Breast Cancer: Evidence-Based Medicine." *Clinics* 66(12): 2133–39.

Nowacki,M., Janik,P., and Nowacki, P. (1996). "Inflammation and Metastases." *Medical Hypotheses* 47(3): 193–96.

Patel, S., and Goyal, A. (2011). "Recent Developments in Mushroom as Anti-Cancer Therapeutics: A Review." *3 Biotech* 2(1): 1–15. Published online November 25, 2011. doi: 10.1007/s13205-011-0036-2.

Perocco P. (2006). "Glucoraphanin, the Bioprecursor of the Widely Extolled Chemopreventive Agent Sulforaphane Found in Broccoli, Induces Phase-I Xenobiotic Metabolizing Enzymes and Increases Free Radical Generation in Rat Liver." *Mutation Research* 595(1): 125.

Raghvendra, M. S., Singh, S., Dubey, S. K., Misrad, K., and Khare, A. (2011). "Immunomodulatory and Therapeutic Activity of Curcumin." *International Immunopharmacology* 11(3): 331–41. http://www.sciencedirect.com/science/article/pii/S1567576910002687?via%3Di hub.

Schmidt, M., Pfetzer, N., Schwab, M., Strauss, I., and Kämmerer, U. (2011). "Effects of a Ketogenic Diet on the Quality of Life in 16 Patients with Advanced Cancer: A Pilot Trial." *Nutrition & Metabolism* 8(1): 54. doi:10.1186/1743-7075-8-54.

Sharma R. A., Steward W. P., and Gescher A. J. (2007). "Pharrmacokinetics and Pharmacodynamics of Curcumin." In *The Molecular Targets and Therapeutic Uses of Curcumin in Health and Disease*, edited by B. B. Aggarwal, Y. J. Surh, and S. Shishodia. Boston: Springer.

Skerrett, P. J. (2014). "Selenium, Vitamin E Supplements Increase Prostate Cancer Risk." Harvard Health Blog. https://www.mayoclinic.org/diseases-conditions/prostate-cancer/in-depth/prostate-cancer-prevention/ART-20045641.

Tallmadge, K. (2013). "Understanding the Power of Omega-3s." (Op-Ed). Livescience.com. https://www.livescience.com/38477-omega3-superstars.html.

Tang, N., Wu, Y., Zhou, B., Wang, B., and Yu, R. (2009). "Green Tea, Black Tea Consumption and Risk of Lung Cancer: A Meta-Analysis." *Lung Cancer* 65(3): 274–83.

University Of North Carolina at Chapel Hill. "UNC-CH Study Offers New Evidence That Garlic Protects Against Cancers." ScienceDaily, October 4, 2000. http://www.sciencedaily.com/releases/2000/10/001004072443.htm.

Wong, K., Tse, S., Wong, L., Leung, C., Fung P., and Lam, W. (2004). "Immunomodulatory Effects of *yun zhi* and *danshen* Capsules in Health Subjects: A Randomized, Double-Blind, Placebo-Controlled, Crossover Study." *International Immunopharmacology* 4(2): 201–11.

Yin, Z., Fujii, H., and Waishe, T. (2010, December). "Effects of Active Hexose Correlated Compound on Frequency of CD4+ and CD8+ T Cells Producing Interferon-γ and/or Tumor Necrosis Factor-α in Healthy Adults." *Human Immunology* 71(12): 1187–90.

Zaini, R., Brandt, K., Clench, M., and Le Maitre, C. (2012). "Effects of Bioactive Compounds from Carrots (Daucus carota L.), Polyacetylenes, Beta-Carotene and Lutein on Human Lymphoid Leukaemia Cells." *Anticancer Agents in Medicinal Chemistry* 12(6): 640–52. (Formerly *Current Medicinal Chemistry - Anticancer Agents*). https://www.researchgate.net/publication/283715462_Effects_of_Bioactive_Compounds_from_Carrots_Daucus_carota_L_Polyacetylenes_Beta-Carotene_and_Lutein_on_Human_Lymphoid_Leukaemia_Cells.

Zhou, S., Kachhap, S., Sun, W., Wu, G., Chuang, A., Poeta, L., Grumbine, L., Mithani, S. K., Chatterjee, A., Koch, W., Westra, W. H., Maitra, A., Glazer, C., Carducci, M., Sidransky, D., McFate, T., Verma, A., and Califano, J. A. (2007). "Frequency and Phenotypic Implications of Mitochondrial DNA Mutations in Human Squamous Cell Cancers of the Head and Neck." *Proceedings of the National Academy of Sciences of the United States of America* 104(18): 7540–45. doi:10.1073/pnas.0610818104.

Zuccoli, G., Marcello, N., Pisanello, A., Servadei, F., Vaccaro, S., Mukherjee, P., and Seyfried, T. N. (2010). "Metabolic Management of Glioblastoma Multiforme Using Standard Therapy Together with a Restricted Ketogenic Diet: Case Report." *Nutrition & Metabolism* 7(1): 33. https://doi.org/10.1186/1743-7075-7-33.

CHAPTER 5:
INTEGRATIVE TREATMENT PLANS IN ACTION

Chen, N. (2008). "Prolonged Metronomic Chemotherapy in Advanced Non-Small-Cell Lung Cancer Is Associated with Excellent Long-Term Survival." *Clinical Lung Cancer* 9(5): 290.

Chen, Q., Espey, G., Krishna, C., et al. (2017). "Pharmacologic Ascorbic Acid Concentrations Selectively Kill Cancer Cells: Action as a Pro-Drug to Deliver Hydrogen Peroxide to Tissues." *Proceedings of the National Academy of Sciences of the United States of America* 102(38):13604–609.

Cimminoelli, L. (2017). "Function Blocks Aberrant Self-Renewal and Leukemia Progression." *Cell* 170(6): 939–55.

Creagan, T., Moertel G., O'Fallon, R., et al. (1979). "Failure of High-Dose Vitamin C (Ascorbic Acid) Therapy to Benefit Patients with Advanced Cancer: A Controlled Trial." *New England Journal of Medicine* 301(13): 687–90.

Kang, D., Weaver, M., Park, N., Smith, B., and McArdle, T. (2010). "Significant Impairment in Immune Recovery Following Cancer Treatment." *Nursing Research* 58(2): 105–14. doi:10.1097/NNR.0b013e31818fcecd.

Kang, H., Kim, B., Piao, C., Lee, K., Hyun, J., Chang, Y., and You, H. (2013). "The Critical Role of Catalase in Prooxidant and Antioxidant Function of p53." *Cell Death and Differentiation* 20(1): 117–29. Published online August 24, 2012. doi:10.1038/cdd.2012.102.

Kerbel, R. S. (2014). "Development and Evolution of the Concept of Metronomic Chemotherapy: A Personal Perspective." In *Metronomic Chemotherapy*, edited by G. Bocci and G. Francia. Berlin, Heidelberg: Springer.

Mauri, D., Kamposioras, K., Tsali, L., Bristianou, M., Valachis, A., Karathanasi, I., Georgiou, C., and Polyzos, P. (2010). "Overall Survival Benefit for Weekly vs. Three-Weekly Taxanes Regimens in Advanced Breast Cancer: A Meta-Analysis." *Cancer Treatment Reviews* 36(1): 69–74. doi:10.1016/j.ctrv.2009.10.006.

Pignata, S., et al. (2013). "A Randomized Multicenter Phase III Study Comparing Weekly versus Every 3 Weeks Carboplatin (C) Plus Paclitaxel (P) in Patients with Advanced Ovarian Cancer (AOC): Multicenter Italian Trials in Ovarian Cancer (MITO-7)—European Network of Gynaecological Oncological Trial Groups (ENGOT-ov-10) and Gynecologic Cancer Intergroup (GCIG) trial." ASCO 2013, Abstract LBA5501. https://www.medpagetoday.com/meetingcoverage/asco/39612.

SEER 18 2007-2013, All Races, Females by SEER Summary Stage 2000. https://seer.cancer.gov/statfacts/html/breast.html.

CHAPTER 6:
MOVING FORWARD WITH INTEGRATIVE CANCER TREATMENT

Brahmer, J., et al. (2015). "Nivolumab versus Docetaxel in Advanced Squamous-Cell Non–Small-Cell Lung Cancer." *New England Journal of Medicine* 373(2): 123–35.

Galon, J. (2006). "Type, Density, and Location of Immune Cells within Human Colorectal Tumors Predict Clinical Outcome." *Science* 313(5795): 1960–64.

Herbst, S., Prager, D., Hermann, R., Fehrenbacher, L., Johnson, B., Sandler, A., et al. (2005). "A Phase III Trial of Erlotinib Hydrochloride (OSI-774) Combined with Carboplatin and Paclitaxel Chemotherapy in Advanced Non-Small-Cell Lung Cancer." *Journal of Clinical Oncology* 23(25): 5892–99.

Hodi, S., et al. (2010). "Improved Survival with Ipilimumab in Patients with Metastatic Melanoma." *The New England Journal of Medicine* 363(8): 711–23.

Kalathil, S., Lugade, A., Miller, A., Iyer, R., and Thanavala, Y. (2013) "Higher Frequencies of GARP+CTLA-4+Foxp3+ T Regulatory Cells and Myeloid-Derived Suppressor Cells in Hepatocellular Carcinoma Patients Are Associated with Impaired T-Cell Functionality." *Cancer Research* 73(8): 2435–44. http://www.cancer.gov/about-cancer/treatment/research/car-t-cells.

Pardoll, D. (2012). "The Blockade of Immune Checkpoints in Cancer Immunotherapy." *Nature Reviews Cancer* 12(4): 252.

Pasquier, E., Kavallaris, M., and André, N. (2010). "Metronomic Chemotherapy: New Rationale for New Directions. *Nature Reviews Clinical Oncology* 7(8): 455–65.

Patel, S., and Kurzrock, R. (2015). "PD-L1 Expression as a Predictive Biomarker in Cancer." *Immunotherapy Molecular Cancer Therapeutics* 14(4): 847–56.

Rosell, R., et al. (2012). "Erlotinib versus Standard Chemotherapy as First-Line Treatment for European Patients with Advanced EGFR Mutation-Positive Non-Small-Cell Lung Cancer (EURTAC): A Multicentre, Open-Label, Randomised Phase 3 Trial." *Lancet* 13(3): 239–46.

Tokheima, C., Papadopoulosc, N., Kinzlerc, K., Vogelsteinc, B., and Karchin, R. (2016). "Evaluating the Evaluation of Cancer Driver Genes." *Proceedings of the National Academy of Sciences of the United States* 113: 14330–35.

INDEX

ABOUT THE AUTHORS

Nick N. Chen, MD, PhD is the founder and medical director of the Seattle Integrative Cancer Center in Seattle, Washington. He is a board-certified medical oncologist and internist with a PhD in immunology. He is a member of the American Society of Clinical Oncologists (ASCO) and the International Society of Integrative Oncology (SIO). He is a pioneer in the clinical application of metronomic low-dose chemotherapy and integrative oncology in the management of advanced cancers with over fifteen years' experience treating cancer patients with both conventional chemotherapy and immunotherapy modalities. Dr. Chen also has trained and practiced medicine on three different continents, which has afforded him extensive knowledge of different treatment models, many of which he incorporates into his practice. This broad spectrum of treatment options offers immense benefits for his patients. The Seattle Integrative Cancer Center (SICC) is an integrative cancer treatment facility where innovative and cutting-edge oncology, such as metronomic low-dose chemotherapy, immunotherapy, and gene-targeted therapy are integrated with supportive naturopathic oncology, nutrition, and other complementary therapies. Patients at SICC often describe it as "out of box" or "ahead of the curve" for the relentless effort of its staff to provide the best comprehensive treatment approaches in the world.

David Tabatsky is a writer, editor, teacher, and performing artist. His publications include *Reimagining Women's Cancers: The Celebrity Diagnosis Guide to Personalized Treatment and Prevention* (2016), coauthored with Michele Berman and Mark Boguski; and *Reimagining Men's*

Cancers: The Celebrity Diagnosis Guide to Personalized Treatment and Prevention (2016), with Mark Boguski and Michele Berman; *Write for Life: Communicating Your Way through Cancer* (2013); *Chicken Soup for the Soul: The Cancer Book: 101 Stories of Courage, Support and Love* (2009), coauthored with Jack Canfield, Mark Victor Hansen, and Elizabeth Bayer; editor of Elizabeth Bayer's *It's Just a Word* (2009); *Dear President Obama: Letters of Hope from Children across America* (2009), coauthored with Bruce Kluger; *The Boy Behind the Door: How Salomon Kool Escaped the Nazis* (2009), coauthor with Sanford Batkin; *The Intelligent Divorce: Taking Care of Your Children* (2009, 2010), coauthored with Mark R. Banschick; and *The Wright Choice: Your Family's Prescription for Healthy Eating, Modern Fitness and Saving Money* (2011), with Randy Wright, MD. David also was consulting editor for Marlo Thomas for her *New York Times* bestseller *The Right Words at the Right Time, Volume 2: Your Turn* (2006).